# Hand Reflexology: A text book for students

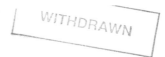

*The hands of those I meet are dumbly eloquent to me. The touch of some hands is an impertinence. I have met people so empty of joy that when I clasped their frosty fingertips it seemed as if I were shaking hands with a north-east storm. Others there are whose hands have sunbeams in them, so that their grasp warms my heart.*

Helen Keller

# Hand Reflexology: A text book for students, second edition

## Kristine Walker

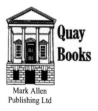

Quay
Books

Mark Allen
Publishing Ltd

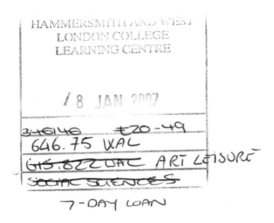
Quay Books Division, Mark Allen Publishing Limited, Jesses Farm,
Snow Hill, Dinton, Salisbury, Wiltshire, SP3 5HN

British Library Cataloguing-in-Publication Data
A catalogue record is available for this book

© Mark Allen Publishing Ltd 2002
ISBN 1 85642 208 9

Printed in the UK by Cromwell Press, Trowbridge, Wiltshire

346146

# Contents

# Foreword

Kristine Walker's teaching, research and clinical practice in the field of hand reflexology has been exceptional. In this revised edition of *Hand Reflexology: A text book for students*, she brings knowledge and insights coupled with extremely clear and informative illustrations. I was fortunate to meet Kristine at a European reflexology conference several years ago and since then she has become an immensely approachable colleague who is always willing to share her knowledge in an intelligible and understandable manner.

I first heard of Kristine's pioneering work with hand reflexology many years ago and was fascinated to discover that foot and hand reflexology were equally effective in helping to trigger the body's innate healing response. It was Kristine I turned to for advice as I developed and researched new techniques in Vertical Reflex Therapy (VRT). I had discovered that the reflexes became extra sensitive and responsive when the hands and feet were treated in a weight-bearing position. Most reflexology courses give only cursory attention to the hand reflexes but her specific work on hand reflexology is invaluable to me, especially when I work the hands and feet simultaneously. Many reflexology text books have little information on the hands and I always recommend Kristine's book and charts to my students.

*Hand Reflexology: A text book for students* can be enjoyed at many levels and will be extremely useful to the professional reflexologist, to other complementary therapists and to lay people who want some easy to learn self-help techniques.

It is a privilege to work and teach with Kristine on joint weekend courses and to benefit from her extensive knowledge, her sense of humour and teaching skills. This book is the result of hard work, inspiration and dedication and deserves to be a success.

Lynne Booth
February 2002

# Introduction

Since the publication of the first edition of *Hand Reflexology: A text book for students*, I have continued to use hand reflexology on my clients as part of their reflexology sessions and teach it to students and laymen. It has been useful for demonstration purposes when explaining to groups of people the theories and practice of reflexology, and as my knowledge of the subject continues to grow I have been able to add to my presentations new and exciting information. Over the years I have become more and more convinced that zone therapy, as discovered by William Fitzgerald, holds the key to greater understanding of this subject, and this is where my focus has been.

Although this book was written for students, I have had a number of telephone calls, letters and e-mails from people new to reflexology who were able to follow the text and give themselves or their partners a satisfactory treatment with good results. With this in mind, I have updated some of the information in the book while keeping the practical information the same so that it is still easy to follow and use.

I am gratified to find that since the first edition was published in 1996, subsequent reflexology books by other authors have given credit to the practice of hand reflexology. This is a great step forward from the days when it was considered to be for self-treatment, that the treatment was not very effective, and that the hands were not as sensitive as the feet — all of which I had discovered was not the case.

However new you are to this subject, I think you will be surprised by its effectiveness even if carried out in an amateur and ham-fisted way. I am continually delighted by the results I achieve through this therapy, and regularly discover new and interesting ways to apply and use it, and of course, the more I use it, the better I get! I hope that you enjoy *Hands* as much as I have.

Kristine Walker
February, 2002

# 1

# Reflexology

This chapter includes:

- the background to reflexology
- the principles of reflexology
- the charts that help to explain reflexology
- the supporting theories of reflexology.

## The background

Most books about reflexology describe how ear, nose and throat specialist, Dr William Fitzgerald (1872–1942), developed zone therapy in the United States early this century. It is not clear where he discovered the principles, although he may have come across them during a visit to Europe around 1902, where a number of manuscripts had been recently published about zones and pressure point work. There is a history of working on the feet in many cultures, both in the East and the West and, although his sources appear to be Western, the origins are felt to lie within the thousands of years of Eastern traditions which include clinical massage and acupuncture.

Fitzgerald discovered that if pressure was applied to the nose, throat and tongue, sensations in particular areas were deadened. This could be extended to produce pain relief by exerting pressure over bony areas of the hands and feet and also other joints of the body. He began to map out these areas systematically, noting conditions associated with them. This is what he termed 'zone therapy'. He divided the body into ten zones and discovered that, by working in a zone, everything in that zone would be affected (*Figure 1.1*). Unlike the pathways of the Chinese meridian system, these zones are complete segments of the body set out as five longitudinal slices beginning on either side of the medial line, and beginning and ending in the top of the head, the fingers and the toes.

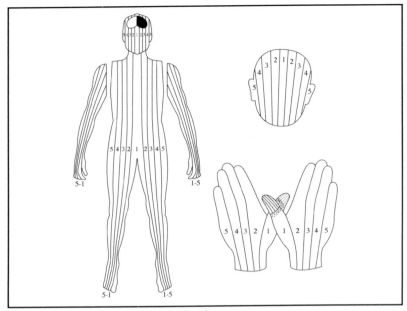

**Figure 1.1: The ten zones**

Dr Joe Shelby Riley of Washington DC used and refined zone therapy and added eight horizontal divisions to the zone chart (*Figure 1.2*). He developed a way of working with specific points by using a hooking technique of the thumb and fingers instead of the various items of equipment, such as metal combs and rubber bands, that Dr Fitzgerald had used to aid the application of pressure.

Dr Riley's therapist, Eunice Ingham, at first called this 'compression massage', later naming it 'Reflexology'. Eunice Ingham used a technique of alternating pressure which she found to have a stimulating effect on specific parts of the body. Her work was developed on the feet and charts were drawn with the help of her niece, Eusabia Messenger, showing the reflexes to specific areas, parts and functions of the body on the feet. These charts have changed very little since that time and are used by reflexologists today (*Figure 1.3*). As the charts have been copied or redrawn, or when an overlap with the reflex points has been found to occur with the acupressure points on the meridian system, some slight variations in the charts have occurred, but the majority of the points have remained constant. Dwight Byers, nephew of Eunice Ingham, has said that after twenty years of investigating the variations, he has found that the most accurate chart is the original one.

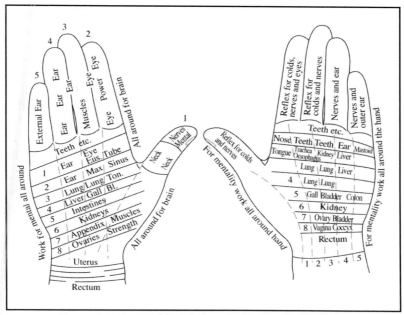

**Figure 1.2: Copy of hand chart by Dr Joe Shelby Riley**

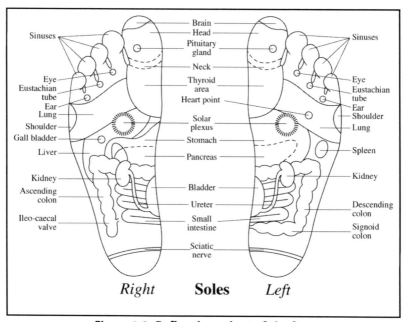

**Figure 1.3: Reflexology chart of the feet**

Eunice Ingham's pioneering work and teaching in foot reflexology was brought to England by Doreen Bayly in 1966. Perhaps because feet are proportionally larger than hands and it is always easier to learn and locate the reflex points on the feet, the hands have been somewhat neglected in England. You will find that these points on the hands are easily located (*Figure 1.4*), and the hands are just as sensitive as the feet, and in some cases, even more so. Although this book sets out to teach hand reflexology, it is my belief that both the hands and the feet should be worked to obtain maximum benefit, as reflexologists in the United States continue to do, and ways of doing this will be discussed in a later chapter.

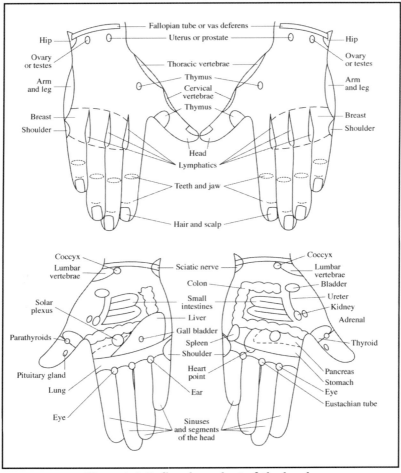

**Figure 1.4: Reflexology chart of the hands**

# Supporting theories — how does reflexology work?

## The nervous system

Nobody knows how information about one part of the body can present itself at an extremity for us to assess with our fingertips, but there are some clues as to how pressure on one part of the body can stimulate a response in another area or organ. In the late 1880s, John Hughlings Jackson, Sir Henry Head, Sir Charles Sherrington and others interested in this work formed the Neurological Society of London in order to encourage the pooling and exchange of ideas about all aspects of the brain and nervous system.

In 1893, Sir Henry Head developed an idea of John Hughlings Jackson (1835–1911) that the nervous system consisted of layers, each restrained by the layer above. With the help of patients with traumatic lesions of the spinal cord, Head was able to chart areas according to the spinal segment to which it belonged. He found that the whole body and limbs could be marked into areas which correspond to the distribution of pain given off from one segment of the spinal cord. Head eventually established areas of skin sensitivity associated with diseases of the internal organs and produced a chart known as 'Head's zones', which was later developed as dermatomes (*Figure 1.5*). He proved that there was a neurological relationship between the skin and the internal organs of the body.

Sir Charles Sherrington (1860–1952) proved that stimuli are produced within the organism by movement in its own tissue, known as proprioception. In 1906, he wrote a book which explains how the brain, spinal cord and numerous reflex pathways respond and adjust to internal or external stimuli. Today we have an understanding of what we could call our sixth sense, or kinaesthetic sense. We receive information from sensory nerve endings in bone and muscle tissue and combine this with the information received from the other senses to give us specific details of our position in space, how each part is arranged in relation to all the other parts of ourselves, and the level of tension in each muscle at any given time. By exposure to sensory stimulation of a specific kind on a regular basis, we can increase this awareness and begin to make changes to ourselves and our bodies.

Around the same time in other parts of the world, similar discoveries were being made. In Germany Dr Alfons Cornelius found that pressure to certain parts of the body, possibly working within nerve pathways, triggered mental and physical response, such as variation in temperature and moisture, and changes in blood pressure.

There are over 7,000 nerve endings in the feet and as many in the hands. It seems possible that their stimulation would lead to responses and adjustments elsewhere in the body.

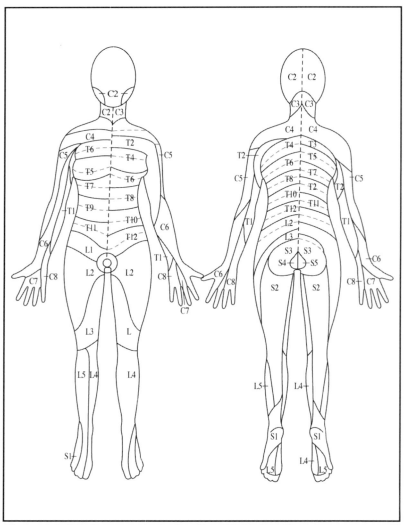

**Figure 1.5: Head's zones were developed into dermatomes — an area of skin supplied by a single spinal nerve**

# Relaxation

In everyday living, we need a certain amount of stress in order to function. Without this we would sit back and allow the world to pass us by without achieving anything. Stress stimulates the production of adrenaline, noradrenaline and cortisol to effect a number of physical changes in the body that we know as the 'fight or flight' response — increased pulse rate and blood pressure, rapid breathing, muscle tension, perspiration, cessation of digestive processes and an increase of blood sugar — all in preparation for action. Some people experience this effect frequently, and some people become addicted to it. When this becomes a normal state of being, then the body begins to suffer. The kind of symptoms which start to manifest are headaches, nausea, indigestion, insomnia, nervous tics, stammering and loss of confidence. The long-term effects might lead to more chronic conditions, such as high blood pressure, heart attacks, ulcers, migraine and nervous breakdown.

A short period of relaxation will often allow a break in this pattern, long enough to review the factors that stimulate this response. With the mind calmed by soothing massage, reflexologists often find that clients are able to make decisions about changes in their lives that are long overdue, or at least comprehend the reasons for the state in which they find themselves. Clients often report that they are 'more able to cope' after a reflexology treatment.

According to Hans Selye, the body adapts to physical stress. When the reflexologist applies a pattern or sequence of pressure, the body begins to relax because its stress pattern is temporarily interrupted or diverted. Muscles held in a state of tension as a protective device begin to relax. Digestive juices begin to flow more easily, breathing becomes deeper and the circulation of blood and lymph improves. Reflexology is said to 'normalise' bodily functions, inducing a state of homeostasis.

# Endorphin release

When we experience pain, endorphins are released, those neuro-transmitters that act like morphine. Pressure is also linked to endorphin release. Strong tactile stimulation, such as pressure, diminishes pain through competition as the signals alerting the brain to pressure compete with those signalling pain, jamming the lower nerve bundles in the central nervous system and causing more stimulus than the system can interpret. The result is an anaesthetic effect.

## Touch

The power of touch has been recognised universally and for a very long time. In the Ebers Smith Papyrus, which dates from the earliest period of Egyptian history, the most common phrase referred to the use of hands in therapy. We know that physical contact is crucial during the early stages of life. In the Far East people go for a massage because they feel like it. It makes them feel good, and when you feel good you are in a better position to fight the effects of stress and ill-health. In the West, physical contact has very much fallen out of favour, to the extent that people are almost afraid to comfort or touch anyone outside their immediate family group for fear of accusations of improper behaviour. And yet we are told that a hug a day from someone we like stimulates the production of T-cells, that are so important to the immune system and releases melatonin, a mood-enhancing chemical. Animals introduced into homes for the elderly are said to have added a new dimension to the lives of the residents who are able to experience the tactile sensations of stroking and holding. Stroking or being stroked reduces blood pressure and improves the flow of blood and lymph through the capillaries.

Many people are deprived of the touch of another. It is no wonder that people living alone, in particular the elderly, are so enthusiastic about reflexology.

## Holism

One of the characteristics of traditional Chinese medicine is a belief that the part contains the whole. Chinese doctors have believed for thousands of years that there are maps of the entire person on various parts of the body that can be used for diagnosis and treatment. These maps are called homunculi or little men, and are thought to be found on the ears, face, eyes, nose, hands and feet. Some modern Chinese doctors have even found homunculi on the metacarpal bone attached to the index finger and on the femur of the upper leg. The sensory cortex of the brain reflects the homunculus.

Holographic photography is a way of converting two-dimensional photographs into a three-dimensional illustration. If a laser is shone through one part of the image, the entire image can be reproduced. Similarly, if the holographic plate is shattered, each piece will show, not a fragment, but the image in its entirety.

In the holistic or holographic model of reflexology we do not need to find a direct link between a part of the body and the hand or the foot, because the connection is a correlation between the overall pattern of the hands or feet and the overall pattern of the body. By manipulating the pattern on the hand we can alter the body pattern. If the microcosm reflects the macrocosm, then each cell will contain the common pattern and the information about the whole body would be reflected therein. Stimulation of the cell or group of cells will bring about change elsewhere.

## The meridians

From ancient China comes the Tao (pronounced 'dow'), based on a flow of energy expressed in two forms (yin and yang) which balance every aspect of creation, known as Ch'i. In the body, a blockage in this flow creates ill-health and Chinese medicine is based on its correction. Ch'i is said to flow in channels, linking organs and ending in the fingers and toes. Pressure on these endings would clear the meridians and stimulate a good flow of Ch'i (*Figure 1.6*).

## Chakras

Therapists who work with chakras trace ill-health to the poor functioning of chakras (meaning 'wheels'). Major ones are thought to be placed where the meridians cross each other twenty-one times; minor ones where they cross fourteen times, and forty-nine lesser points where the meridians cross seven times. Beyond this, there are many tiny force centres which may correspond to the acupuncture points of Chinese medicine. The major ones bring Ch'i into the meridian system and are again related to organs and the glands of the endocrine system. These may become damaged by traumatic accident or emotional shock. Minor chakras are found in the centre of the palms.

## Healing

After many rigorous trials, healing continues to increase in popularity. Healing techniques are based upon four simple concepts:

❖ That we are composed of energy which vibrates at different rates and links the physical body with the mind, the emotions and the spiritual self.

❖ Disease stems from imbalance in this system.

❖ When two or more people come together, some kind of energy is exchanged between them.

❖ That there are sources of energy outside the body that can be utilised to improve our health and vitality.

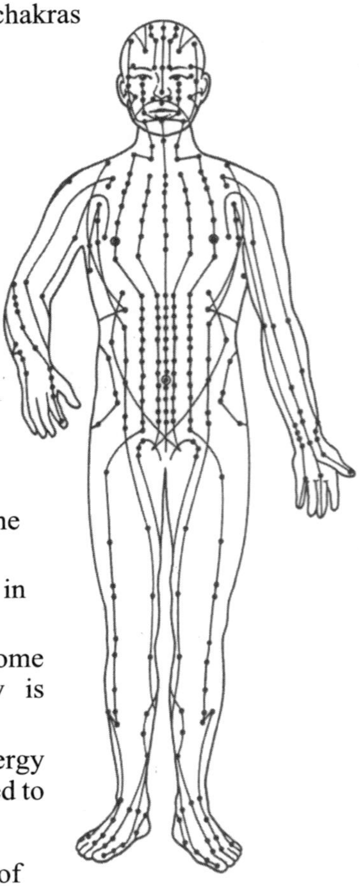

There may well be some kind of energy exchange between the reflexologist and the client and, in the United States, science graduates are trying to construct a machine to measure this exchange. At present it seems that the better the relationship, the more the healing processes are activated. Healers also feel that they can channel incoming energy through themselves and into another person to correct imbalances in the energy system. Laying on of hands, or some kind of physical contact, is often employed. Reflexologists often notice the increase in the temperature of the hands when giving a treatment, and sometimes the 'tingling' sensations experienced by healers.

**Figure 1.6: The meridians**

# Placebo

The placebo effect and psychosomatic phenomena indicate that the mind affects body function quite dramatically. If the mind is convinced that health will ensue by swallowing a pill or receiving therapy then it often will, but a mental vote of no confidence is likely to hold things up. According to the television programme 'Pulse', shown in January 1996 on Channel 4, British television, 'Heart Sink' patients are the one in five patients visiting a general practitioner that nothing seems to help. These patients' problems seem to be a mixture of a physical condition and an emotional one, and they feel their body pain as a result of their emotional state, the most common being known as TATT (Tired all the time). Groups that fall into this category appear to be the elderly, single mothers, the homeless, people living alone and low income groups. Depression seems to have an adverse effect on physical well-being, and psycho-neuroimmunology studies this kind of effect. It is likely that good therapists are effective in eliciting the placebo response, and all healthcare professionals are in a position to utilise this healing effect as, indeed, many do.

# Natural recovery

The body will naturally move towards good health providing that there is nothing to stop it, and the best 'cures', conventional or otherwise, are the ones which trigger nature into doing all the work. Without any intervention there is likely to be improvement of common, everyday complaints, and a measure of the effectiveness of a therapy like reflexology has to show that results go beyond this. Like the placebo effect, a gentle nudge by the therapist to stimulate the client's innate healing capacity, the *vis medicatrix naturae*, may well be the most important, if often underlying, aspect of any healthcare treatment.

Today, there are theories and practices linking many of the therapies with reflexology — shiatsu or acupressure techniques facilitate Ch'i flow by pressure on points of the body, polarity therapy (*Figure 1.7*) balances energy flow and zero balancing works on a model of vertical pathways through the body. Focusing, hypnotherapy and neuro linguistic programming all work to bring about an inner shift in consciousness that frees the body of its patterns of pain and ill-health. The connection between all alternative and complementary therapies is the stimulation of the healing processes through the co-operation between therapist and client.

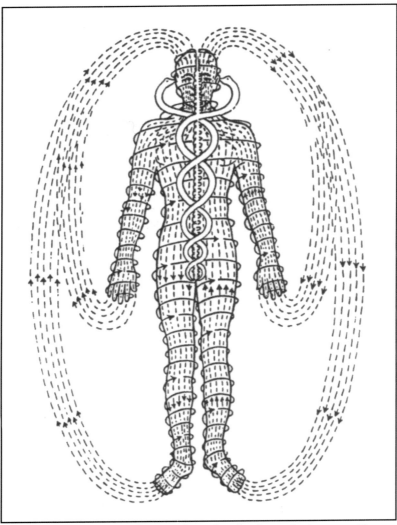

**Figure 1.7: Polarity therapy chart showing how electromagnetic currents flow around and through the body**

# 2

# Before you start

This chapter includes:

- observation skills
- listening skills
- record cards
- safety
- major drug groups.

Right from the first moment your client enters your therapy room, you will be concentrating on him/her. Your answer phone should be switched on and the 'Do not disturb' notice should be hung on the door. This is the client's time, the client's hour of relaxation, the client's hour of your undivided attention. As a therapist you are required to have a broad overview of the client and an awareness of the factors that might affect his/her health. A consultation must take place in order to uncover this information; skill and sensitivity must be developed in order to do this in an appropriate and inoffensive way. The client must be asked if you may write down personal details and, if necessary, it should be explained that these details will help you to decide on the length and frequency of treatment or whether you are able to offer help at all.

## Observation skills

These are one of the most important skills that you must develop as a therapist.

You will not, of course, make any judgement about what you see; neither will you attempt any diagnosis. What you observe will help you to decide as to the degree of ill-health that your client is suffering and your plan of action. If your client looks radiant, then your treatment will help to keep him or her this way. The following is a list of the things that you might notice about your client:

⌘ Posture — is the body upright or unbalanced?

⌘ Gait — is the body flexible and fluid?

⌘ Complexion — does the skin colour look good?

⌘ Skin — is it free of spots or blemishes; is it dry or greasy?

⌘ Eyes — are they clear and bright?

⌘ Hair — is it dull or thinning, oily or with dandruff?

⌘ Nails — are they bitten, chipped, flaking or discoloured?

⌘ Body odour — is this unusual or offensive?

⌘ Manner — is this confident, reticent, nervous or vague?

## Listening skills

Much more information can be obtained if we develop our listening skills. How often do we listen to people but we don't really hear what they are saying? We may even misinterpret the message — people do not always tell you exactly what they mean. If you do not understand what is being said then ask for clarification, particularly if medical terms that you may not have come across before are introduced. Make sure that the body language matches what is being said and listen carefully to the inflexions and intonations in the voice. Someone telling you how relaxed he/she is while sitting on the edge of a seat and speaking with a high, squeaky voice does not equate. Listen for the following:

⌘ Is the voice shrill, hurried, breathless or strangled?

⌘ Is it hesitant, low and quiet?

⌘ Does the client stammer, unable to find the right words or finish sentences?

⌘ What are the underlying emotions?

Look for signs, such as dull and monotonous tones, frequent swallowing or a quaver in the voice, or while your client is speaking watch for hand wringing, crossed arms and eye contact. We see these actions and signals every day in the people with whom we associate and this determines how we react and interact with them. As therapists, we can empathise with our clients, acknowledging pain, injury, illness or discomfort without allowing our own thoughts, feelings or prejudices to become apparent and influence the way that we treat our clients. As professionals, we try to relate to everyone we see in the same way. When we listen, we try to focus on the content and meaning and absorb a sense of the 'message' that the client is trying to get across. We are not waiting for our turn to speak, nor are we thinking of suitable comments to make. We do not tell the client about ourselves unless it is a means of giving information relating to him/her or his/her own condition.

## Record cards

Having gained the above information we are now ready to fill out a record card. It is important to keep records for each client so that you can monitor the treatment's progression and remind yourself at each session which areas have been given special attention and which areas need to be checked for changes at the next session. The card is the property of the client and the information it contains should be confidential unless you are instructed by him or her to pass it or the information to someone else. Steps should be taken to ensure that the card is destroyed in the event of your death.

The following should be recorded:

| | |
|---|---|
| Name | Address and telephone number |
| Occupation | Date of birth |
| Doctor's details | Present problem |
| Illnesses | Accidents |
| Operations | Medication |
| General state of health | General observations |
| Date of first session | Recommendations |
| Results of first session | |

### Why are all these details needed?

The name, address and telephone number are necessary for identification and in case you need to change an appointment or send information to your client. The date of birth will give you information as to his/her phase of life. Both the phase of life and occupation can affect the state of health of the client. The doctor's details are required in case it becomes necessary to advise him or her that you are giving reflexology to one of his/her patients. If, in your opinion, a client is presenting with an untreated or undiagnosed serious medical condition, ask the client to see a general practitioner as soon as possible. The client can, if necessary, make another appointment to see you at a later date.

The presenting problems are the reason for the visit by the client. Sometimes there will not be any such problems as reflexology is a prophylactic treatment, ie. it helps to prevent problems, and many people enjoy this period of relaxation for its own sake rather than because they are suffering from an illness. You may also like to ask why the client has chosen reflexology which will help you to discover what his/her expectations are and if you are the right person from whom he/she should be seeking help. Accidents, illnesses, operations and medication will give you a clue as to where sensitive areas on the hand may be found, and if you need to take special care. Although reflexology is thought to be totally safe we need to apply commonsense to certain situations, and there may be occasions when we feel that we need to have clearance from the client's doctor before proceeding.

At this stage it is unnecessary to record minor conditions experienced in the past as this may take up too much time. What you are looking for is anything that might be affecting the current state, such as car accidents, debilitating illnesses, major surgery and chronic complaints.

## Safety

### Conditions where reflexology is contraindicated

It would not be wise to treat someone with a contagious disease, with undiagnosed severe pain or internal bleeding, particularly if there is a possibility of pregnancy. In all such cases referral to a doctor should be immediate.

## Conditions when care should be taken

### Diabetes

Diabetics who are used to regulating their own insulin levels often do not consider themselves to be ill. Your guide should be the condition of the skin. In diabetics, fragile or thin skin may tear and flesh may bruise easily leading to ulceration and further problems, so caution is necessary. If the client complains of numbness or tingling in the fingers, ask them if they have been checked for diabetes.

### Deep vein thrombosis, phlebitis or acute inflammation of the venous or lymphatic systems

Obtain the doctor's permission. As a 'rule of thumb', I avoid any condition which involves acute severe inflammation of the tissues until it has been diagnosed and treated by a medical doctor. The 'healing crisis' experienced by some clients after a treatment, in which symptoms worsen before they get better, may cause further problems.

### Osteoporosis

Great care should be taken with fragile bones. There is greater risk of this disease as we grow older, so lighter treatments are always recommended for the elderly.

### Wounds, scars and bruises

Avoid wounds and do not work on areas that might cause undue pain or discomfort to your client.

### Herpes zoster (shingles)

Reflexology may aggravate the condition further while in an active phase. Wait until an attack has cleared before you treat.

### Epilepsy

It is possible that your client may have a fit during treatment. Discuss the possibility before treatment and, if you both feel comfortable about handling the situation should it arise, then go ahead. Case studies show that the incidence of fits is reduced in some people after a course of reflexology.

### Children

Short, light treatments are best.

### Following surgery

Research shows that reflexology can help the body to recover more quickly but a light treatment should be given for two weeks after surgery, avoiding the reflex to the site of the surgery for the first week.

## Major drug groups

### Medication

The type of medication that your clients have been prescribed will tell you a great deal about their condition. Some drugs will mask the responses that you expect when pressing sensitive points on the hands. Reflexology seems to work well with most allopathic and natural medicines and remedies, but check your list of cautions and, if in doubt, ask the doctor's permission to work on his/her patient. Some drugs can cloud the judgement and prevent clear thought; others produce side-effects, such as nausea, insomnia, vomiting or constipation that no amount of reflexology will be able to relieve. When a diabetic client is taking insulin, he/she must be able to regulate insulin intake as the function of the pancreas may improve with treatment. If you intend to become a professional reflexologist, a guide to medicine and drugs will help you to identify the system or systems in need of attention, the severity of the condition and the side-effects that may be experienced.

The major drugs groups are as follows:

| | |
|---|---|
| *Brain and nervous system:* | analgesics |
| | anti-anxiety |
| | antidepressants |
| | antipsychotic drugs |
| | anticonvulsant drugs |
| | antiemetics |
| | nervous system stimulants |
| | sleeping drugs |
| | drugs for migraine |
| | drugs for Parkinson's disease |
| *Respiratory system* | bronchodilators |
| | decongestants |
| | drugs to treat coughs |

| | |
|---|---|
| *Vascular system* | digitalis<br>beta blockers<br>vasodilators<br>diuretics<br>anti-arrhythmics<br>anti-angina drugs<br>anti-hypertensive drugs<br>lipid-lowering drugs<br>anti-blood clotting agents |
| *Digestive system* | antacids<br>anti-ulcer drugs<br>anti-diarrhoeal drugs<br>laxatives<br>anti-inflammatories<br>drugs for rectal and anal<br>    disorders<br>drugs for treating gallstones |
| *Muscular and skeletal systems* | anti-inflammatories<br>anti-rheumatics<br>corticosteroids<br>muscle relaxants<br>drugs for bone disorders<br>drugs for gout |
| *Allergy* | antihistamines |
| *Infections and infestations* | antibiotics<br>antibacterials<br>anti-virals<br>vaccines and immunisations<br>anti-fungals<br>anti-malarials<br>anti-protozoal drugs<br>anti-tuberculins |
| *Endocrine system* | corticosteroids<br>drugs for diabetes<br>drugs for thyroid disorders<br>drugs for pituitary disorders<br>male and female sex<br>    hormones |

| | |
|---|---|
| *Malignant and immune disease* | anti-cancer drugs<br>immunosuppressants<br>AIDS/HIV drugs |
| *Genito-urinary system* | drugs of menstrual disorders<br>oral contraceptives<br>drugs for infertility<br>drugs used in labour<br>drugs for urinary disorders |
| *Skin* | anti-pruritics<br>topical corticosteroids<br>drugs for acne and psoriasis<br>anti-infections<br>sunscreens<br>drugs to treat parasites |

The general state of health of your client and your general observations may include diet, exercise and lifestyle, as well as emotional and mental states. I emphasise 'general' as I feel that the taking of the medical history should not take more than fifteen to twenty minutes and should not be intrusive. More personal details will emerge as you build up your relationship with your client, possibly over a period of weeks.

The details of your sessions can be brief, outlining the condition of the hands, sensitive or painful areas and points that feel too hard, soft, gritty etc. Your recommendations would be the frequency of treatment sessions or referral to a GP or another practitioner if appropriate. At the next appointment you would find out how the client felt following the previous session, particularly if there was any reaction to the treatment (see 'Healing crisis', *Chapter 6, p.77*) so that you can modify the current session, and if there is any improvement in the presenting problem. These details from session to session will show the progress that is being made and the changes in the hands as conditions improve. I prefer to make notes at the end rather than during the session, so that I do not lose contact with the client's hands until the treatment has finished.

# 3

# The treatment

This chapter includes:

- seating
- assessment
- opening movements
- grips and supports
- working techniques
- the sequence
- closing movements.

## Seating

Before you begin, study the anatomy of the hand in *Chapter 5* (*Figure 5.2*), and the hand reflex chart in *Chapter 1* (*Figure 1.4*). It is important that both you and your client are seated comfortably during the reflexology session. If you have a massage couch or reclining chair, sit to one side facing your client, working with the hands on a covered pillow placed on the client's lap. You should be able to work easily on the hands with the minimum amount of movement for you and your client during the session. Make sure that your own chair is the right height and close to the side of the client.

Another way to work is for you to sit facing each other with a pillow resting on your knees between you, or by using a narrow, padded table. Neither you nor your client should have to lean further forward than is easy or comfortable.

Hand reflexology can be carried out successfully sitting next to someone on a bus, train, aeroplane or cross channel ferry and is useful for help in relieving travel sickness. It can be carried out equally well standing up. Hands are easily accessible and treatment can be given in almost any situation. In this book, the treatment I describe is carried out with the therapist facing the client. For learning purposes, it is better to start by using a small table with a cushion or padding on the top, covered with a clean towel. Several folded towels would do. You can place this book to one side so that you can follow the instructions as you work. If the hand to be treated is sticky, use a little unscented baby powder. If you are used to using oils for foot reflexology, then do so on the hands if you wish, although the techniques described in this book will have to be adapted to the way that you work.

## Assessment

Start your session by placing the client's hands palms down on the pillow and making a visual and tactile **assessment** of them. When you wish to turn a hand over, sandwich one between your own two hands and turn. You will find that you can only turn one way. A healthy person will have hands that are a good colour with good skin and muscle tone, pleasantly warm but without dry or excessively moist skin, and nails will be in good condition with lustre. You are looking for clues that might tell you that all is not well, but without coming to any conclusions about the state of health unless relevant information has been given while you were taking the medical history. Watch for injuries that may cause discomfort if touched, or for swollen, painful joints. The following is a hands check list:

⌘ Skin condition — dry, cracked, thin or callused.

⌘ Temperature — hot or cold or variations between the fingers and palms.

⌘ Colour — mottled, pale, red, yellow or blue-tinged.

⌘ Hydrosis — slightly wet or extreme perspiration.

⌘ Tone — firm, flabby, strong, flexible or stiff.

⌘ Nails — split, flaked, broken, pale or blue tinged; they may be ridged or spotted.

⌘ Shape — are the fingers straight or bent; are the tips bulbous; are you able to flatten the palms?

Make a note of relevant findings on the medical card and record changes that take place from session to session as the client's health improves.

## Opening movements

Having noted the above, you are now ready to do some opening movements before you begin the sequence. You and your client should remove watches and jewellery. As the hands are used in normal everyday activities and are fairly flexible, it is not necessary to perform much in the way of relaxing movements. Before starting the treatment some initial contact of a soothing nature will help to relax and reassure the client. The client's hand should be palm down on the cushion.

❖ Take the right hand in both of yours, thumbs on top and, with the thumbs parallel and touching in the centre of the dorsum, slide out to the sides, gently opening out the metacarpals. Gently pull and rotate each of the fingers and thumb in turn and place them on the cushion. Sandwich the hand between your own and turn the hand over so that the palm faces up.

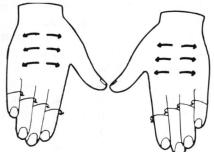

❖ Support with your right hand and place the fingertips of your left hand to the fingertips of your client. Stroke up the hand and lower arm, skin to skin, almost to the elbow, and then stroke back down to the hand sliding off the thumb and slightly pulling it, in one continuous, fluid movement. Repeat three times.

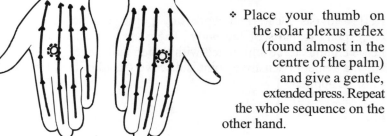

❖ Place your thumb on the solar plexus reflex (found almost in the centre of the palm) and give a gentle, extended press. Repeat the whole sequence on the other hand.

**Figures 3.1a/b: Opening movements**

The client may now remove the left hand from the cushion and we can begin on the right. There is no reason for starting on the right side — if you wish, you could start with the instructions for working on the left hand. When you are familiar with the reflex points and the techniques, you could work from hand to hand or from system to system.

## Grips and supports

The way you support the hands is very important. Unlike the feet, the hands will not stand up on their own so you have to make sure that you have full control as you work. Remember too, that your client can see everything that you are doing. With practice you will soon give a confident and assured treatment. Generally, the hand is cupped in your palm, client's palm up, with your thumb steadying on the palmar side. When working on the dorsal side this is not as comfortable, so steady the hand by supporting the wrist from underneath, or holding firmly while allowing it to rest on the cushion. When you apply pressure, even lightly, it is necessary to have the resting fingers or a thumb of the working hand on the other side of the client's hand so that some leverage can be applied. Avoid gripping too firmly on this side or the client may feel discomfort in an area where you are not intending to work.

## Working techniques

Reflexologists locate and work tiny points on the hands which correspond to parts of the body. There are several thousand tiny nerve endings to be stimulated with thumb and finger pressure, and when a tender or sensitive point is discovered, additional techniques must be applied.

### One

For working large areas of the hand, use the thumb or finger walking technique. Locate a point on the tip of the thumb to which you can apply pressure without straining the thumb joint, and press an area the size of a pin head. Let the thumb joint be slightly bent. Pressure with a straight thumb is poor technique and will not allow you to creep forward from point to point. Every time you press, imagine that you are making a connection with the corresponding point in the body as if turning on a light switch. After pressing one point, extend your thumb a little so that you can move very slightly forward to apply pressure once again to the next point. Continue in this way, moving forward in tiny creeping movements, making positive connections with the skin with every movement. Make sure the movement is away from the wrist, and not back towards it. The same technique can be used with the fingers. Sometimes your pressure will be firm, sometimes light, depending on the sensitivity of your client and the area that you are working.

## Two

When a point is sensitive, press into the point for about twelve seconds, then release. Repeat this three times. You may wish to go back to this point once or twice during the session in order to relieve the sensitivity further, balancing the reflex and its corresponding body part or function. This method is used to relieve pain in the body as it has an anaesthetising effect on the corresponding body part.

## Three

Rotation of the point is another way of working specific reflex points When contact is made with the thumb or finger, the point is massaged in a small rotating movement for a few seconds.

When the skin of the hand is very slack, and the thumb or finger walk is impossible to carry out, then this method is a good alternative.

## Four

To access some of the points a hook back technique is required. Press into the point with the thumb and hook it back towards your palm, almost getting 'under the skin'.

## The sequence on the right hand

### Working the thumb — the head and neck reflexes

Start with the client's palm facing up and the hand resting on the cushion. Grip the thumb with your left hand and use your right thumb to work from the tip to the base of the thumb, covering one side. Change hands and work from base to tip on the other side. You will need to do about six rows in all to cover the entire thumb. Work an extra row over the tip of the thumb for reflexes of the brain. The thumb joint represents the teeth. The proximal segment contains the reflexes of the thyroid and parathyroid, so work in this area well looking out for skin texture resembling medium grade sand paper, often found in people with a thyroid imbalance. The reflex of the pituitary gland is found in the centre of the thumb, often in the centre of the fingerprint whorl. Use the hooking technique, pushing from under the point and up into it, or hook up from above.

### Working the fingers — segments of the head, and sinuses

Support the fingers with your left hand and start working the little finger with your right thumb. Work each segment thoroughly with three or four rows of thumb-walking before moving on to the next segment. Move across to the ring and middle fingers, then change hands for the index finger. Turn the hand over, and work the dorsal side of the fingers, massaging the joints as you come to them. Turn the hand back to the palmar side. Locate the ear reflex with your thumb between the little finger and the ring finger, the eustachian tube reflex between the ring finger and the middle finger, and the eye reflex between the middle finger and the index. Press firmly into these points, working them as described in sections two and three of 'Working techniques' if the client experiences discomfort (*Figure 3.2*).

### Finger pads — The lungs and cardiac area

Support the hand with your left hand, client's palm up, and use your right thumb to massage each pad of the metacarpophalangeal joint, and in between (*Figure 3.3*). This is a difficult area to execute a thumb walk, so each pad has to be worked independently. Use a small rotation of the thumb in one spot before moving on to the next point to repeat the movement. Work from the little finger to the index finger.

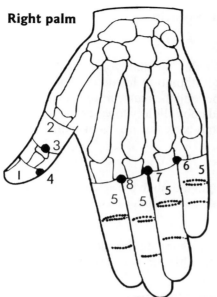

**Right palm**

1. Brain
2. Thyroid
3. Parathyroid
4. Pituitary
5. Sinuses
6. Ear
7. Eustachian tube
8. Eye

**Figure 3.2: Reflexes of the head and neck**

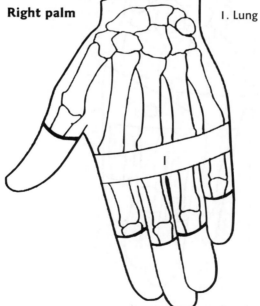

**Right palm**

1. Lung

**Figure 3.3: Reflexes of the lung**

## The palm — the digestive system

### *Gall bladder*

Still working with the palm up and your left hand supporting underneath, use your right thumb to locate the gall bladder reflex. This point is found just beyond the metacarpophalangeal joint of the fourth finger. Press in and hook slightly towards the little finger. You will be pulling your thumb back towards your palm (see 'Working techniques', section 4, *p. 25*).

### *Liver*

Thumb walk with your right thumb in the area shown in the diagram. Approach and work from several directions.

### *Stomach and pancreas*

Continue to work this area, changing the support hand and working thumb if it is more comfortable for you. Two to three rows should cover this area (*Figure 3.4*).

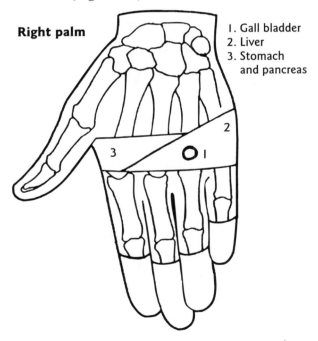

**Right palm**

1. Gall bladder
2. Liver
3. Stomach and pancreas

**Figure 3.4: Reflexes of the digestive system (i)**

## Ileo-caecal valve, ascending and transverse colon and small intestine

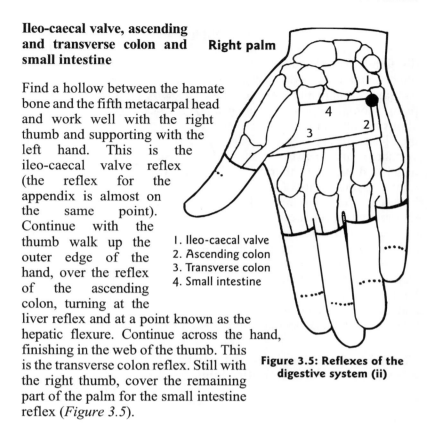

**Right palm**

Find a hollow between the hamate bone and the fifth metacarpal head and work well with the right thumb and supporting with the left hand. This is the ileo-caecal valve reflex (the reflex for the appendix is almost on the same point). Continue with the thumb walk up the outer edge of the hand, over the reflex of the ascending colon, turning at the liver reflex and at a point known as the hepatic flexure. Continue across the hand, finishing in the web of the thumb. This is the transverse colon reflex. Still with the right thumb, cover the remaining part of the palm for the small intestine reflex (*Figure 3.5*).

1. Ileo-caecal valve
2. Ascending colon
3. Transverse colon
4. Small intestine

**Figure 3.5: Reflexes of the digestive system (ii)**

## Bladder, ureter, kidney and adrenal gland

Change the supporting hand and place your left thumb in the centre of the thenar muscle. Work this point for the bladder reflex. Thumb walk to the base of the muscle to pick up the crease or line (palmists call it the life line). Change hands and continue up this line towards yourself. You are working the ureter reflex. Find the kidney point and access it from directly above with firm pressure. This is a difficult point to access correctly, so try on yourself first. Once you have located it, use your left thumb to the left of the kidney point, hooking under the thenar muscle to locate the adrenal reflex (*Figure 3.6*).

## The side of the hand — the spine

Sandwich the hand between yours with the right hand on top. Work with your left thumb down the side of the hand, starting at the distal thumb joint and feeling for the bone under the skin as you work. Continue round the base of the palm, completing the sequence almost in the centre of the wrist at the coccyx reflex. The cervical vertebrae are between the distal and proximal thumb joints, the thoracic between the proximal thumb joint and the head of the first metacarpal, and the lumbar vertebrae between the first metacarpal and the scaphoid bones, with the sacrum and coccyx between the scaphoid and lunate bones (*Figure 3.7*).

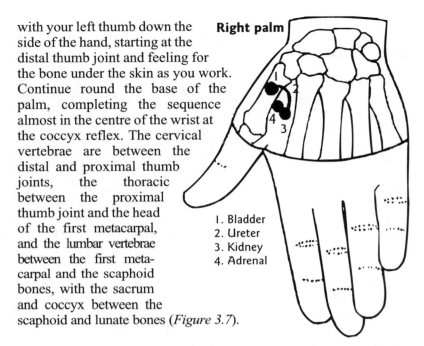

**Right palm**

1. Bladder
2. Ureter
3. Kidney
4. Adrenal

Figure 3.6: Reflexes of the urinary system and adrenals

**The side of the hands — The arm, elbow, knee, leg and sacroiliac joint**

Sandwich the hand again, this time with your left hand on top and working with your right thumb. Thumb walk down the outer edge of the hand, starting at the base of the little finger (the shoulder reflex) carrying on to the centre base of the palm — the sacroiliac joint. The arm reflex is on the fifth metacarpal bone, the elbow and knee reflex at the metacarpal head, the leg reflex over the pisiform and triquetral bones with the sacroiliac joint between the triquetral and lunate bones.

**Across the wrist — The sciatic nerve**

Work across the wrist with a thumb walk, lateral to medial, then change hands and work from medial to lateral. It does not matter with which direction you begin.

Sandwich the hand between yours and turn it over so that the back of the hand faces up (*Figure 3.8*).

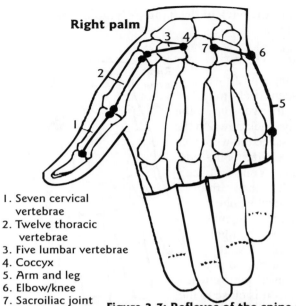

**Right palm**

1. Seven cervical
   vertebrae
2. Twelve thoracic
   vertebrae
3. Five lumbar vertebrae
4. Coccyx
5. Arm and leg
6. Elbow/knee
7. Sacroiliac joint

**Figure 3.7: Reflexes of the spine and
the arms and legs**

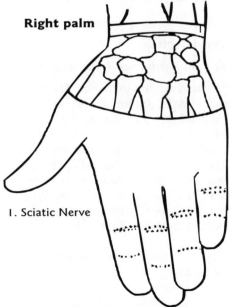

**Right palm**

1. Sciatic Nerve

**Figure 3.8: Reflexes of the sciatic nerve**

## The webs and the back of the hand — lymphatics of the chest and the breast area

### *Breast area*

Use a forefinger to finger walk between each metacarpal from the webs up to the carpals. Slide back down to the web and massage the web. Use your thumb on the palm side for leverage. You will be accessing the area from between the client's fingers.

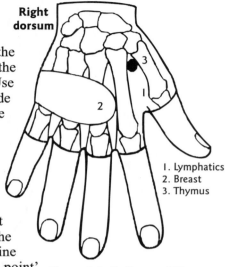

Locate the thymus point with your right thumb and hook it towards the client's thumb. Do not work this point if your client is pregnant, as it is close to the meridian for the large intestine known as the 'bearing down point' (*Figure 3.9*).

**Figure 3.9: Reflexes of the chest**

## The wrist — reproduction

### *Ovary/testes, fallopian tube/vas deferens and uterus/prostate*

These areas are found around the wrist. The ovary/testes point is on the outside of the wrist (palm down) in a hollow between the triquetral and the lunate, and passes through to the palmar side. Rotate the point with your left thumb. Find similar uterus or prostate points on the inside of the wrist between the scaphoid and the radius and work in the same way. The fallopian tube or vas deferens connects the two points between the protruding heads of the radius and ulnar. Use a thumb walk to work this. Work this area, too, for inguinal lymphatics (*Figure 3.10*). Squeeze down the back and sides of the arm for extra stimulation of the reflexes for general reproduction and elimination.

The right hand is now complete and you change to the left, starting with the palm up.

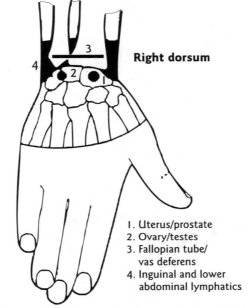

1. Uterus/prostate
2. Ovary/testes
3. Fallopian tube/ vas deferens
4. Inguinal and lower abdominal lymphatics

**Figure 3.10: Reflexes of the reproductive system**

## The sequence on the left hand

### Working the thumb — the head and neck reflexes

Grip the thumb with your right hand and use your left thumb to thumb walk from the tip to the base of the thumb, covering one side. Change hands and work the other side from base to tip. Cover the tip of the thumb for the reflexes of the brain using a thumb walk with the side of your thumb, the joint, to cover the teeth reflexes, the proximal segments for reflexes to the thyroid and parathyroids and the pituitary gland in the centre of the thumb whorl. The parathyroid and pituitary points can be accessed by hooking from above (*Figure 3.11*).

### Working the fingers — segments of the head and sinuses

Support the fingers with your right hand and start working the little finger with your left thumb, one segment at a time, four rows for each segment depending on the size of the finger. Move from finger to finger, changing hands to work the index finger. Turn the hand over and work the dorsal side, not forgetting to massage each joint for specific teeth reflexes. Turn back to the palmar side and locate the ear, eustachian tube and eye reflexes, pressing the points firmly with the side of your thumb (*Figure 3.11*).

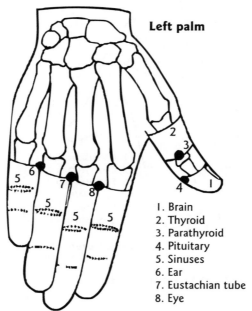

**Left palm**

1. Brain
2. Thyroid
3. Parathyroid
4. Pituitary
5. Sinuses
6. Ear
7. Eustachian tube
8. Eye

**Figure 3.11: Reflexes of the head and neck**

## Finger pads —the lungs and cardiac area

With the client's hand palm up, support with your right hand and rotate each pad at the base of the fingers and between each pad with your left thumb. Work from the little finger to the index finger. Locate the heart helper point on the fourth metacarpophalangeal joint with your left thumb. Allow the hand to fold slightly as you press and hook into the point (*Figure 3.12*).

## The palm — the digestive system

### The spleen

Supporting with the right hand, place your left thumb on the spleen reflex and press using the lateral side of your thumb to hook into the spleen point (see 'Working techniques', section 4, *p. 25*; *Figure 3.13*).

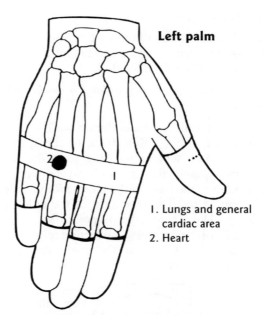

**Left palm**

1. Lungs and general cardiac area
2. Heart

**Figure 3.12: Reflexes of the lung and heart**

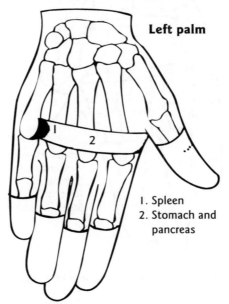

**Left palm**

1. Spleen
2. Stomach and pancreas

**Figure 3.13: Reflexes of the digestive system (i)**

### Stomach and pancreas

From the spleen point, continue with a thumb walk with your left thumb across the stomach and pancreas reflexes, two or three rows depending on the size of the hand.

### Transverse colon, descending colon, sigmoid colon, rectum and small intestines

Change the supporting hand and thumb walk with your right thumb on the transverse colon reflex, back to the spleen point and the splenic flexure. You will be working from the web of the thumb across the hand. Change the support hand and work down the side of the client's hand to the base of the palm with your left thumb, down the descending colon. The next turn of the colon is known as the sigmoid flexure. Work across the sigmoid colon reflex across the base of the palm to finish on the pad at the rectum reflex. Complete working the palm by covering the area of the small intestine reflex with your left thumb (*Figure 3.14*).

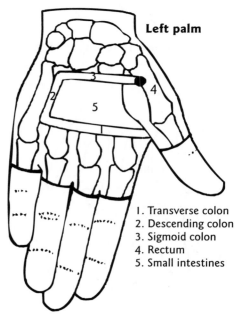

**Left palm**

1. Transverse colon
2. Descending colon
3. Sigmoid colon
4. Rectum
5. Small intestines

**Figure 3.14: Reflexes of the digestive system (ii)**

## Bladder, ureter, kidney and adrenal gland

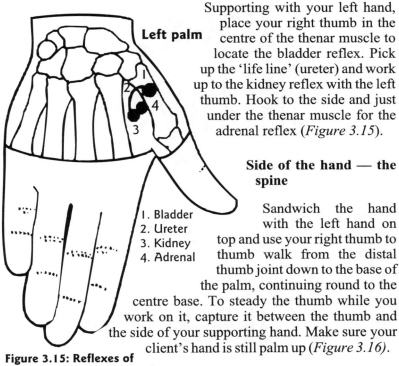

Supporting with your left hand, place your right thumb in the centre of the thenar muscle to locate the bladder reflex. Pick up the 'life line' (ureter) and work up to the kidney reflex with the left thumb. Hook to the side and just under the thenar muscle for the adrenal reflex (*Figure 3.15*).

**Left palm**

1. Bladder
2. Ureter
3. Kidney
4. Adrenal

**Figure 3.15: Reflexes of the urinary system and adrenals**

### Side of the hand — the spine

Sandwich the hand with the left hand on top and use your right thumb to thumb walk from the distal thumb joint down to the base of the palm, continuing round to the centre base. To steady the thumb while you work on it, capture it between the thumb and the side of your supporting hand. Make sure your client's hand is still palm up (*Figure 3.16*).

### The side of the hand — the arm, elbow, knee, leg and sacroiliac joint

With the palm still up, sandwich the hand again with your right hand on top and work down the side of the hand from the base of the little finger, carrying on round to the base of the palm. You should be using your left thumb to do this (*Figure 3.16*).

### Across the wrist — the sciatic nerve

Thumb walk across the wrist from lateral to medial and from medial to lateral, changing thumbs as you change direction. The lines across the wrists are sometimes called 'the bracelets' (*Figure 3.17*). Sandwich the hand and turn it over.

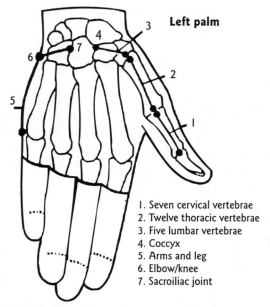

1. Seven cervical vertebrae
2. Twelve thoracic vertebrae
3. Five lumbar vertebrae
4. Coccyx
5. Arms and leg
6. Elbow/knee
7. Sacroiliac joint

**Figure 3.16: Reflexes of the spine, arm and leg**

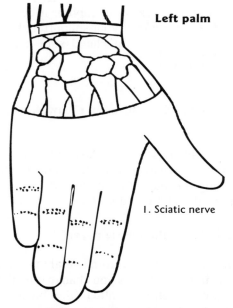

1. Sciatic nerve

**Figure 3.17: Reflexes of the sciatic nerve**

**The webs and the back of the hand — the lymphatics of the chest and breast area**

Use a forefinger to finger walk between each metacarpal to the carpals and draw back down to the web each time, finishing with massaging the web. Approach this area from between the fingers. Locate and work the thymus point with your left thumb and with the hooking technique (*Figure 3.18*).

**The wrist — reproduction**

Locate, press and rotate with your right thumb the ovary/testes point in the hollow between the triquetral and lunate bones, and the uterus/prostate point between the scaphoid and head of the radius with your left thumb. Join the two points across the wrist between the heads of the radius and ulna for the fallopian tube/vas deferens reflexes, and thumb walk around this area for the inguinal lymphatic reflexes. Squeeze down the sides and back of the arm for extra stimulation of the areas for general reproduction and elimination (*Figure 3.19*).

The sequence is now complete and you may wish to return to areas that were sensitive or felt as if they needed some extra stimulation. To complete the treatment carry out further relaxing movements.

## Closing movements

Return to the right hand and place it palm down on the cushion. Bend your fingers and with your thumb underneath the hand massage into the wrist area. Now make a cup with one hand and place it on the top of the knuckles. Make a fist with the other and place it underneath on the palm. Massage the cupped hand with your fist with a small circular movement. Because your client's hand is in between, the joints will be rotated and loosened. Do both these movements on the left hand and then turn both hands over.

Touch fingertips with your client and carry out the same movement that you used for the opening but with both hands at the same time — stroking up the arms and back down to the hand, pulling off down the thumbs. Do this three times.

Place both thumbs on the solar plexus points, one on each hand. Instruct your client to breathe in. With each 'in breath' press the points and with each 'out breath', release. Repeat three times. Not only is this a lymphatic pump but it also helps to wake up the client. Reflexology often sends the client to sleep.

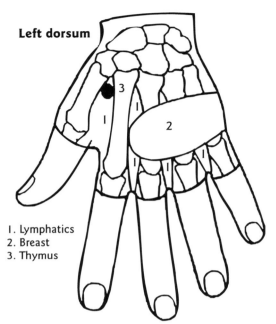

**Left dorsum**

1. Lymphatics
2. Breast
3. Thymus

**Figure 3.18: Reflexes of the chest**

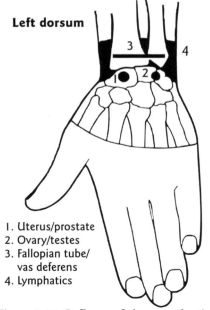

**Left dorsum**

1. Uterus/prostate
2. Ovary/testes
3. Fallopian tube/
   vas deferens
4. Lymphatics

**Figure 3.19: Reflexes of the reproductive system**

Allow your client to relax for a few minutes before leaving. If a drink is required make it warm water — never cold — as the body temperature will have dropped. An exception to this rule would be in high temperatures. Discuss any recommendations concerning further treatments and arrange the next appointment. If you are in professional practice, this is when the client will usually pay you. When your client has left, record your observations and findings on the record card.

## The sequence — showing the direction of movement across the hands and listing the points covered

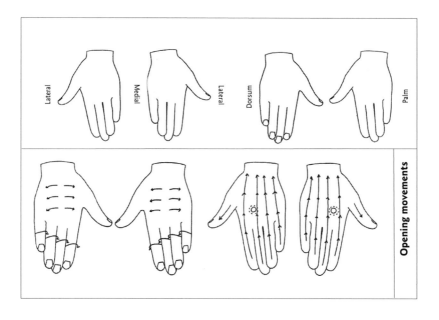

| | |
|---|---|
| head<br>brain<br>teeth<br>jaw<br>thyroid<br>parathyroids<br>pituitary<br>sinuses<br>eyes<br>eustachian tube<br>ears | **The thumbs** |
| | **The fingers** |
| lungs<br>heart<br>gall bladder<br>liver<br>stomach<br>pancreas<br>ileo-caecal valve<br>colon<br>spleen<br>intestines | **The finger pads** |
| | **The palms** |
| bladder<br>ureter<br>kidney<br>adrenals | **The thenar muscles** |

| | |
|---|---|
| cervical vertebrae<br>thoracic vertebrae<br>lumbar vertebrae<br>coccyx | **The lateral palm** |
| arms<br>elbows<br>knees<br>hips<br>sacroiliac joint<br>sciatic nerve | **Medial palm and wrist** |
| lymphatics<br>breast<br>thymus | **The dorsum** |
| ovary/testes<br>uterus/prostate<br>fallopian tube/vas deferens | **The dorsal wrist** |
| | **Closing movements** |

# 4

## The therapist

This chapter includes:

- you, the therapist
- the professional reflexologist
- working on your own hands
- being creative.

### You, the therapist

A client comes to you for help, often in desperation. Although you know that you cannot heal the client, you have an important responsibility. Through the administration of your art you offer treatment to the client, and it is reasonable for the client to expect an improvement in his or her condition. People react to symptoms of illness in different ways. Some people endure discomfort while others immediately visit a general practitioner. Sometimes the appearance or a recurrence of a symptom prompts the visit or perhaps the realisation that others with the same symptoms have been diagnosed and treated. Other factors may prompt the visit, such as interference with lifestyle or career. When people are busy, they do not always pay attention to the signals of the body and it is only at times of rest that they become aware of the problem. Pain experience and attitude varies from culture to culture and some people see health as an exception. Others feel indignant if they are not experiencing a continual glow of good health. In some cases, people only need to have their pain or illness acknowledged and then they can begin to heal. For these people, reflexology may be a 'last resort'. It is intriguing to discover why they have chosen this moment to come to see you.

Can you perceive the needs of your clients clearly? What do they hope to achieve by receiving treatment and what are their expectations? Can you meet their needs? Often naming the condition brings some form of relief and you are not able to do this. Knowing yourself, knowing your limitations and having the confidence to express them indicates a responsible therapist. If we have been taught well, we will have faith in our teacher and our therapy. If we are self-taught, we need to work with many people to judge how effective our therapy can be and be confident in our skills. Regardless of the teaching methods you have chosen, interacting with other reflexologists boosts confidence, while the exchange of ideas and information helps to confirm the benefits of your skills and keeps you up-to-date with current developments, techniques and research. If possible, become a member of a reflexology organisation to gain:

- the security needed to grow
- the stability of clear and definite limits
- the confidence to try new and creative methods
- the help and support of other reflexologists
- enthusiasm and motivation.

Although enthusiasm will carry you a long way, good basic working knowledge, recognised by our clients, will provide greater benefits. Good results will then boost self-esteem and encourage you to trust your own judgement. Frequently, when practitioners have confidence and trust in the feedback received from carrying out a therapy which they know thoroughly, they start to function on a higher intuitive level.

Do not neglect your own self-development because what you have dealt with, or worked through in terms of dealing with life's challenges, mental, emotional or physical, will help you to develop the empathy and understanding required of a good therapist. Whether or not you wish to practise reflexology as a career, your care and consideration when dealing with a client, friend or family member will be appreciated. Prepare the space in which you will be working before the clients arrive; make sure that both yourself and the area are neat and clean, and that the temperature of the room is appropriate for someone at rest. Welcome your clients into the room and make them feel at ease. Explain what you are going to do, the time it will take and what you expect from them. Attention to this kind of detail shows a respect for others, making them feel special and identifying each person as a unique individual who has taken a big step by coming to see you, in an attempt to take responsibility for his or her own health.

Keep up-to-date with current developments in the world of health and medicine by subscribing to health journals and attending lectures, seminars and evening classes held by healthcare professionals or natural health therapists. Study anatomy, physiology and pathology to increase your understanding of the nature of illness and disease. Collect information about allergy, diet, exercise, entertainment, assertiveness or any other subject or matter that improves the quality of life. The more you grow, the more you have to offer.

## The professional reflexologist

To help us to work safely and within the law, reflexology associations usually publish a code of ethics and practice or a set of guidelines within which we can work to maintain a professional approach, and which will help us to define our limits. These are based on the following principles:

- do not prescribe
- do not diagnose
- do not promise cures
- do not discriminate
- do not treat a specific illness
- do not speak disrespectfully of another therapist
- do not work over a client's pain threshold
- respect your client's confidentiality
- make your fees clear before the treatment commences
- adhere to local by-laws.

***Do not prescribe:*** This means that you cannot instruct your client to take any kind of remedy or carry out any action other than reflexology unless you are qualified to give such advice. When you are qualified and insured, the terms of your insurance will be a further guide. One exception may be water and you can offer your client a drink of warm water (cold water sometimes puts people into mild shock after a treatment) which they may accept or decline.

***Do not diagnose:*** Unless you are a medically qualified doctor you cannot diagnose. You can, however, express an opinion about congestion or imbalance as they are indicated on the hand, and which parts of the body these correspond to on the reflexology charts. As the areas overlap, it is unwise to be specific. Place a hand on your own body to indicate to your client the area of congestion to avoid naming an organ, part or function. To do so may cause unnecessary alarm.

***Do not discriminate:*** A professional therapist will respect all religions and political and social views, irrespective of race, colour, creed or sex. If, on the other hand, you feel that reflexology cannot help, you are obliged to say so.

***Do not treat specific illnesses:*** This means not working on specific areas of the hand to effect a cure, unless to bring relief in a first-aid situation. Many reflexologists like to discuss which parts of the hands and feet should be worked on to help medical conditions, but this is working with the symptoms only. Every system of the body makes some kind of contribution to our well-being, therefore every system should be treated. The client's response should be your guide. If the client feels discomfort when an area is pressed, then further work needs to be done in this spot regardless of whether or not it relates to the presenting problem.

***Do not promise cures:*** Although people visit reflexologists because they have heard of the benefits of the treatment for various ailments, or perhaps have read about one of the many research trials being completed at the moment, reflexologists are not at the stage where they can state categorically that the treatment will be of benefit for a particular person. Everyone is different and our responses vary. Five per cent of our clients may receive no benefit. We treat people, not illnesses. Research will and has shown that reflexology has had a beneficial effect on the relief of symptoms of many conditions and this clause may eventually be retracted. Meanwhile, make a point of obtaining this research information and make it available to prospective clients so that they can judge for themselves.

***Do not speak disrespectfully of another therapist and do not work over a client's pain threshold:*** These are self-explanatory and part of our respect for everyone we come into contact with, in or out of our therapy room.

***Respect your client's confidentiality:*** You may hear things that surprise and horrify you, but all the information you receive from a client and his/her record card is confidential. If your client tells you that they are breaking the law or suffering abuse, or even admit to being abusers themselves, then you will find yourself in a very difficult position, and you will need to discuss this with your client.

***Make your fees clear before treatment commences:*** If you are not insured, you will not be charging a fee and your reflexology will be classed as a hobby. If you wish to carry out reflexology as a business, be clear about your charges. You may decide to charge less for pensioners and the unemployed or you may offer a discount for ten sessions. Perhaps you will charge more for your initial consultation. Write down your charges so that prospective clients can consider them before starting treatment.

***Adhere to local by-laws:*** You may need to register your business with your local council or have your place of work inspected. Find out from your town hall. The compliance office of the Inland Revenue also watches for people who advertise services in the area. Working within the law is part of your professional obligation.

As part of your developing awareness of holistic and complementary therapies, you may visit as many therapists as you can afford, or with whom you may exchange treatments, in order to obtain the names and addresses of therapy specialists who you can trust and refer your own clients with confidence.

## Working on your own hands

Client or therapist, hand reflexology is the ideal therapy for self-treatment. You, the therapist, owe it to yourself and your clients to present a picture of good health and this is one way to do it. Work on your hands wherever you might be when you have a moment to spare, or sit and relax in a comfortable position to give yourself a treat. You may wish to instruct your client to work on his or her own hands between treatments to maintain the healing momentum. If you do this, use the chart (*Figure 4.1*) showing the hands for self-treatment, and colour in the areas to be worked. Start with either hand, using the fingers of the working hand to support. To be thorough, follow a simple routine:

❖ Thumb walk from tip to base of each finger and thumb, and all the way round.
❖ Massage the webs and the points between the fingers.
❖ Cover the entire palm and thenar muscle with the thumb of the working hand. Work from beneath the little finger to the thumb.

Change direction and work from fingers to wrist and from wrist to fingers. Press and rotate all points on the palm, stopping to work out tenderness or areas where you feel some discomfort.

❖ Use your thumb or forefinger to work down both sides of the hands.

❖ Use a forefinger to work on the back of the hands. Work up between the metacarpals from the webs, and slide back.

❖ Press and rotate with your thumb all the way round your wrists.

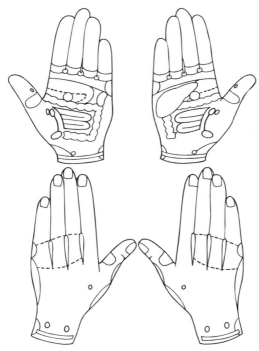

**Figure 4.1: Hand chart for self-treatment**

If your client has long nails, a golf ball or rubber can be used. These are to be used as self-help devices only, not as a method of working on someone else. When using a golf ball, interlace the fingers of both hands and hold the golf ball between the heel of the two hands. Now roll the golf ball, increasing or decreasing the amount of pressure as desired, over your entire palm. Palm to palm, roll the golf ball up and down your fingers. Experiment with a marble, or any ball that you have. Perhaps you have seen 'Chinese Dragon Balls'? These two balls are used as a means of stimulating the meridians in the hands by circling both together round one palm, manipulating them with the fingers. This takes some practise but, like Greek worry beads, once the technique is mastered it is fun to do and extremely soothing. Chinese balls can be bought in gift shops and Chinese supermarkets or grocery stores. A rubber tipped-pencil may be used (rubber end only) to press and rotate into the parts of the hand that you are not able to access with your fingers.

The flexibility of your own hands is important in order to give a good treatment. Because we use our hands so much, we think of them as being flexible, but there are a variety of movements that we do not often utilise, such as rotating the fingers. Crossing the fingers is an example of this. Give your hands a good shake, loosening the wrists and increasing the blood supply to the fingers and nail-beds. Practise playing an imaginary piano to strengthen the fingers. Stress balls or squash balls can be used to strengthen the grip by alternating squeezing and releasing. To increase the sensitivity in your fingertips, run your fingers over a variety of textured surfaces, such as wood grain, brick or knitted fabrics. Like the Princess and the Pea, see if you can locate a piece of thread beneath the page of a book, and then beneath several pages. Then try again, this time with a hair. Spend more time caring for your own hands. After all, they will be on display when you are giving a treatment.

Check how effective your own treatment is by practising on yourself. When you use the thumb or finger walk, do you maintain contact with the skin? Make sure that you do not dig in with your nail. Vary your speed and pressure and feel free to lift your elbow or move your body to make access easier. Relax your shoulders and wrists.

## Being creative

When you are familiar with the sequence and techniques of the hand reflexology treatment, and have practised until it becomes second nature, you can experiment with a variety of ways of working. It's a bit like driving a car — once you have passed your driving test, you can begin to appreciate the car. The art of reflexology is to know when a particular pressure or method is appropriate for a condition or person, and for how long it should be applied. With practice and patience, you can move on from being a reasonable therapist to being a very good one. Many therapists favour one technique and attract people who benefit from this technique as their clients. In the last chapter, I mentioned that when you become confident with your treatment, you start to function on a higher intuitive level. The information you receive when you stop worrying about what you are doing is more subtle. When you work on an area of the hand with sensitive fingertips, you are almost listening to what the hand is telling you it wants you to do. The hand is reflecting the whole body from its own viewpoint, telling the story from the hand's point of view.

First, try working very lightly over an area of the hand, perhaps the fingers. As you lightly stroke each segment allow your fingers to stop and work wherever you feel most inclined to do so. Allow yourself time to probe into the nooks and crannies between bone and flesh, easing out tension. A treatment carried out totally with this sort of pressure seems to affect the emotional and spiritual parts of our being rather than our physical self, and is inclined to send people to sleep. It is a method that I use to shift long-established patterns of ill-health or emotional trauma, sometimes stemming from birth.

Increase your pressure and both you and your client will experience different sensations. You are beginning to probe a deeper layer of tissues and fluids, and making more contact with nerve endings. A brisk and bouncy treatment at this level will make your client feel positive and energised, and is a method I use for people exhausted through stress or illness.

Now work deeply over the bones, not with a thumb walk, but with a constant pressure sliding from joint to joint, ironing out the creases. This is often painful so use it with care and first try it out on yourself. I use this for acute pain and first-aid treatment and I feel it works on deeper physical levels, especially for problems associated with bones and joints.

Experiment with the way that you use your fingers. Sometimes you may feel as if you would like to tap rather than press, to pinch rather than rotate. To access a point deep within the hand, you may want to link palmar and dorsal surfaces with a thumb and forefinger, massaging top and bottom simultaneously, as with the points on the wrist. Try using a thumb and middle finger to link two points that may be connected in some way, such as the reflexes of the top of the head and the base of the spine; or the shoulder reflex and the sixth cervical vertebrae; sense pulses and vibrations or shifts in flow of blood and lymph.

Study the meridian charts and bring pressure on some of these points into your work. Look up diagrams of the nerves of the hand

and find out if pressure on the main nerves is especially painful, and if the points are linked with reflexology or meridian points. Try touching the chakra points on the spinal reflexes and see if you experience any sensations in your fingertips. Meridian and chakra charts can be found in *Chapter 5*. Be as imaginative as you can in your approach and always keep meticulous notes about the treatment that you gave and the responses that you perceived. These different approaches mean that you will never be bored with your reflexology and perhaps you will discover how reflexology works.

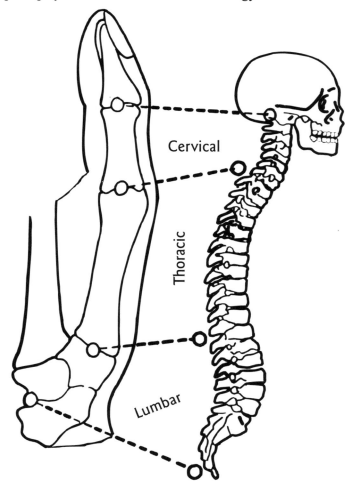

**Figure 4.2: The spinal reflexes on the thumb**

# 5

## All about hands

This chapter includes:

- anatomy
- conditions affecting the hands
- the meridians
- the chakras
- medical palmistry
- chinese fingernail diagnosis
- metamorphic technique
- Jin Shin Jyutsu
- aromatherapy

Although this chapter does not relate directly to reflexology, some knowledge of the way in which hands are used to interpret the functioning of the body may give further insight into the way in which reflexology works. There may be some aspects of these other disciplines which you may wish to include in your treatment, or to study further. As my descriptions are brief, I suggest that for further information you contact experts in these fields, and/or undertake further training or instruction to enable you to utilise the data safely and effectively. Study of the hands is infinite and can take us on many exciting journeys of discovery if we are willing to follow. Reflexology may well be the reference base from which you wish to work, or it may be the springboard into another area for you to explore.

### Anatomy

Hands enable us to grip and manipulate, and are the most versatile part of our body. Muscles in the forearm operate most of the movement in the hands, but short muscles in the palms control the more delicate actions. Humans and other primates are the only creatures to have fingers and thumbs that move independently (the thumbs are 'apposite') enabling the hand to grip. The folds of skin on the tips of our fingers which give us our fingerprints also help us to grip. Man has developed a fine co-ordinated action of the fingers allowing us to adopt a writing position. Nerve endings in our hands provide information, often protective, about our surroundings.

The bones of the forearm, the *radius* and *ulna*, meet at the wrist. When we turn our hand the ulna remains stationary and the distal end of the radius rotates around it, carrying the hand. The head of the radius rotates in the radial notch of the ulna. The wrist, or carpus, is composed of eight carpal bones arranged in two rows of four, named in Latin after the shape they resemble. From below the little finger to the thumb these bones are: proximal row — *pisiform*, *triquetral*, *lunate* and *scaphoid*; and distal row — *hamate*, *capitate*, *trapezoid* and *trapezium*. The radius and the scaphoid form an *ellipsoidal joint*. This type of joint can be flexed or extended and moved from side to side, but rotation is limited.

The skeleton of the palm is composed of five *metacarpal* bones. The proximal base of each one articulates with a carpal bone and the rounded distal head of each one forms the knuckle with its corresponding proximal phalanx. These phalanges in the fingers, proximal, intermediate and distal, form hinge joints with the base of the phalanx in front. At the end of the finger the distal phalanx ends in a tuft which supports the nail. The phalanges are concave on their palmar side because they form the floor of a tunnel roofed by fibrous tissue through which the flexor tendons of the fingers glide in their *synovial sheaths*. The metacarpal of the thumb is short, slight and set freely away from the hand so that it can be opposed to the fingers. There are only two broad phalanges in the thumb.

Most bones develop from cartilage precursors. Ossification is the process by which cartilage is converted into bone as a result of minerals being deposited, especially calcium. Bones do not become ossified until early adult life when bone growth has come to an end. In older people, there may be some bone loss resulting in the thinning of the bones. Flexing a hand to cushion a fall sometimes breaks the end of the radius and occasionally the tip of the ulna, and damage to the scaphoid is not uncommon. Elderly people with thin bones and whose balance is unsteady are particularly susceptible.

Muscles of the hand cannot be disassociated from those of the forearm which are divided into two main groups of flexors and extensors, with their associated nerve trunk. The superficial flexors of the forearm include the superficial flexors of the fingers and the flexors of the wrist joint. The deep flexors of the forearm include the deep flexors of the fingers and the long flexor of the thumb. Between them is the median nerve. The extensor of the forearm also has superficial and deep layers, the main nerve being the radial. The groups of extensor muscles are the extensors of the wrist joint, the extensors of the fingers, which have one tendon each except for the fourth and fifth fingers which have two, and the extensors of the joints of the thumb. All these tendons are bound down by a ligament at the wrist to prevent them from bow stringing backwards, called the *retinaculum*. The palm is bounded by muscles called the *thenar* and *hypothenar* eminences on each side. Between the metacarpals are the *interossei*, the small muscles of the hand.

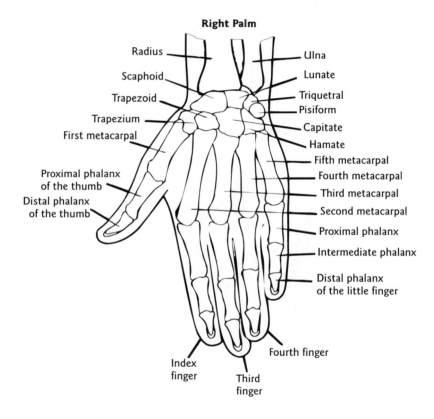

**Figure 5.1: Bones of the hand**

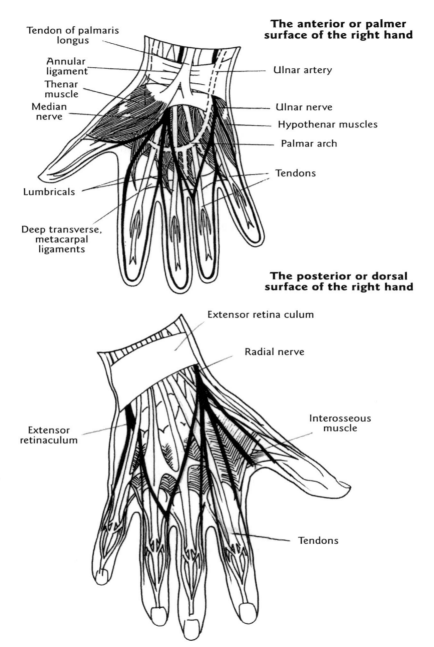

Tendon of palmaris longus

**The anterior or palmer surface of the right hand**

Annular ligament

Thenar muscle

Median nerve

Ulnar artery

Ulnar nerve

Hypothenar muscles

Palmar arch

Tendons

Lumbricals

Deep transverse, metacarpal ligaments

**The posterior or dorsal surface of the right hand**

Extensor retina culum

Radial nerve

Interosseous muscle

Extensor retinaculum

Tendons

**Figure 5.2: The anatomy of the hand**

At the elbow, the brachial artery divides into radial and ulnar branches which run down each side of the forearm. At the wrist, the *ulnar artery* continues into the palm, while the *radial artery* turns on to the back of the carpus to form the dorsal arterial arch. In the palm, there are two arterial arches formed between branches of the two vessels and from these smaller channels lead to the fingers. The veins form a fine network in the hand and forearm, but the lateral or cephalic vein and medial or basilic veins emerge at the elbow. The tiny capillaries are important for temperature regulation. The fine lymphatic vessels correspond to the venous pattern but with the main lymphatic trunks running with the brachial artery entering the main group of lymph glands of the arm in the axilla.

The skin consists of two parts, the epidermis and the deeper connective tissue layer of the dermis. The epidermis on the palms of the hands is very thick to protect these surfaces from wear and tear. The dermis is thin and has its *papillae* arranged in parallel lines to form papillary ridges. The epidermis over this layer reflects this pattern, the basis of fingerprints. Thick skin has numerous sweat glands, the ducts of which open at the summit of the ridges, and there are no hair follicles. Collagen fibres give strength to the skin and the elastic nature of the skin on the back of the hand is due to elastin fibres. This can be demonstrated by lifting the skin away from the back of the hand. When it is released it resumes its original position. If the skin is cut, retraction of the elastin fibres causes the wound to gape.

The nail is a translucent keratin plate embedded in folds of skin. It is free at the tip but, elsewhere, it is firmly attached to the underlying epidermis. Nail growth, which is quicker at the fingers than at the toes, occurs in the nail bed — the epidermis under the fold at the base and sides of the nail is supplied by blood vessels which give them their pink colour. Nails are made of keratin, a hard, fibrous protein, which is also the main constituent of hair.

## Conditions affecting the hands

### Carpal tunnel syndrome or repetitive strain injury (RSI)

Caused by existing arthritis, wrist fractures, thyroid deficiency or fluid retention and, more controversially, by compression of the median nerve through repetitive movement — reflexology has been known to bring relief to this painful condition. The retinaculum divides the hand from the wrist and creates a narrow space, the 'carpal tunnel', through which the median nerve passes to serve the muscles in the hand and give sensation in the fingers. Compression of the nerve can blunt sensations, cause loss of power in wrist muscles and pins and needles in the hand, especially at night. There is often numbness and pain in the thumb and middle finger. Inflammation of the tendons (tendinitis) or the tendon sheath (tenosynovitis) may occur when there is excessive friction between the tendon's outer surface and an adjacent bone. Hand reflexology can help this condition if both thumbs are used simultaneously to push from the edges of the wrist to the centre, relieving the pressure on the median nerve, and thumb walking up the arm to the elbow. Attention needs to be given to the shoulder reflexes.

## Osteoporosis

After middle age, bones become notably thinner and more porous, causing loss of bone mass in both sexes. Falling oestrogen levels in women after the menopause can lead to this with the deposited minerals broken down much faster than they can be formed, thus weakening the bone. The decline in testosterone in men is gradual and they suffer less osteoporosis. Exercise and diet may help to prevent the loss of calcium salts. Reflexology carried out on people suffering from this condition should be very gentle indeed.

## Osteoarthritis

Unlike rheumatoid arthritis which affects several body systems at the same time, osteoarthritis may affect a single joint. Degeneration of the joint may be the result of 'wear and tear', or by cartilage defect, injury or infection. A mild form affects many people over sixty years old due to the erosion of cartilage. The bone surfaces rub together causing pain and inflammation in the joint. Drugs can reduce the inflammation and control the pain to help maintain joint mobility and minimise deformity. Hand reflexology can help to keep this mobility if applied with care, and can be used to help in the prevention of further deterioration.

## Rheumatoid arthritis

This autoimmune form of arthritis develops when the immune system begins to attack body tissues. The joints become inflamed, swollen, stiff and deformed, usually to the same degree on both hands. Stiffness is often worse in the mornings. Reflexology given gently and regularly can help to mobilise the fingers, to relieve pain and boost the immune system function.

## Rashes

Rashes are areas of skin inflammation or groups of spots. They may occur in small patches or cover a large part of the hand. Eczema refers to various skin inflammations with common features which may include itching, red patches and small blisters, and may be an indication of an allergy. Psoriasis is a non-infectious skin disease of unknown cause. The skin has bright red or pink patches with silvery, scaly surfaces. Infectious rashes, such as measles, rubella and chicken pox have a toxic effect on the skin that produces a characteristic, temporary rash. It is unlikely that anyone with a rash on their hands would elect to go for hand reflexology treatment but, should this situation arise, offer foot treatment as an alternative. Reflexology can help stimulate the flow of lymph and stimulation of the capillaries, and may help to improve the immune system function. Do not treat a person with a contagious or undiagnosed condition.

## Vitiligo

This is the absence of cells that produce a dark pigment in the skin called melanin, causing colour irregularity in certain areas.

## Diabetes

Diabetes mellitus is a condition in which the lack of the hormone insulin prevents the body from using the energy generated by carbohydrates. The condition causes a sugar loss in the urine. Diabetics are more liable than other people to develop skin infections, painless ulcers and the arteries and peripheral nerves are prone to degeneration. This often improves with medical treatment. Research has shown that reflexology stimulates the functioning of the pancreas. The hands should be worked gently, to avoid bruising the skin.

## Parkinson's disease

This is a degenerative condition of the brain that occurs more often in men than in women over the age of sixty years. The disease causes weakness and stiffness of the muscles, and interferes with speech and movement. There is often tremor of the hands when they are at rest.

## Raynaud's disease

Hypersensitivity to cold of the arteries supplying the fingers results in restricted flow to this area. The fingers become white and cold to the touch.

## Ganglion

Sometimes a small, painless lump, about the size of a pea, develops in the wrist, caused by swelling in a joint capsule or a tendon. Left alone, it frequently disappears without medical treatment.

## Dupuytren's syndrome

Shrinkage of the fibrous tissue on the palm of the hand causes clawing of the ring and little fingers.

## Iron deficiency (anaemia)

Caused by deficiency of iron, $B_{12}$ and folic acid, haemorrhage or disease. A clinical feature is spoon-shaped nails with a typical hollowing of the centre.

## Warts

A contagious but harmless skin growth caused by the human papilloma virus. Cover with a plaster before you work on the hands.

# The meridians

In many countries, study of the meridians forms an important part in the training of reflexologists. Ch'i is the name for the life-force or subtle energy that permeates the Universe and sustains all living things. In India it is known as Prana, in Japan as 'Qi'. One long, continuous flow moves Ch'i in one direction around the body, circulating twenty-five times a day and twenty-five times a night. An illness is said to be the result of an imbalance in this flow. The channel is separated into fourteen branches or meridians, governed by an organ or function and named after it, although this relationship is as much symbolic as physical. The twelve major meridians have surface and deep pathways with connecting channels between them. On the surface level, they form a continuous loop with the end of one flowing into the beginning of the next, so forming a related pair. Each pair is also bilateral, which means that they follow the same route on each side of the body. The twelve main pairs consist of one yin and one yang meridian which balance each other, and if there is a problem with one, then the other will be affected. Yin energy flows from the feet to the torso, and from the torso along the inside of the arm to the fingertips. Yang energy runs from the fingertips to the face along the back of the arm, and from the face to the feet. It is possible to work on the surface branches of the meridians with touch techniques in order to clear them, and there are various indications which might suggest that a meridian is not functioning as well as it might, thus taking the form of skin disorders, joint problems, blemishes, lumps, bumps or nail problems along the path of the meridian. As hand reflexologists, we are in a good position to study and work on the meridians that are located in the hands and nails. The medical history combined with a good knowledge of the meridians would give us an insight into the functioning of each channel, and our thumb and finger techniques would help to clear blockages. Generally speaking, pressure applied to the meridians is more intense and searching than the reflexology finger or thumb walk. In addition to working directly on the meridian terminals, we would be working on the reflexes to the entire meridian system. The meridians located in the arms and hands along with indication of their imbalances are as follows:

### Thumb — lung meridian (Yin)

Watch for pain or stiffness in the shoulder or elbow joints, carpal tunnel syndrome, tenosynovitis, arthritis in the thumb, warts and spots or ridges in the thumb nail.

### Index finger — the large intestine meridian (Yang)

Nose bleeds, herpes simplex (cold sores) on the lips, throat problems, frozen shoulder, tennis elbow, greasy skin, problems in the index finger and its nail.

### The middle finger — the circulation or pericardium meridian (Yin)

Swollen axillary glands in the armpits, carpal tunnel syndrome, hot palms and problems in the middle finger and its nail

### The ring finger — the triple warmer or endocrine meridian (Yang)

Look for ear and eye problems, shoulder pains, stiffness and pain along the wrist and arm, and problems in the ring finger, such as arthritis or eczema, or its nail.

### The little finger (palmar aspect) — the heart meridian (Yin)

Speech defects, swollen axillary glands, inner arm problems, angina, weak wrists, stiffness, pain or whitlow in the little finger or problems with the nail.

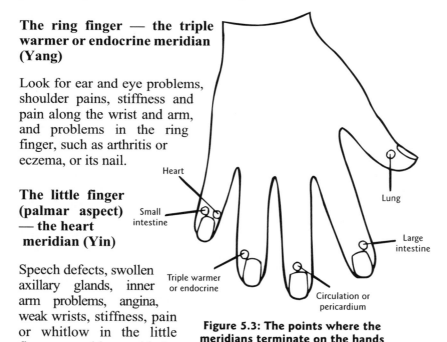

**Figure 5.3: The points where the meridians terminate on the hands**

### The little finger (dorsal) — the small intestine meridian (Yang)

Tinnitus, deafness, trigeminal neuralgia or Bell's Palsy, swollen glands in the neck, aching or stiffness in the shoulder blade, tennis elbow, weak wrists, problems with the little finger or white spots and ridging of its nail.

# The chakras

*Chapter 1* described how the chakras are placed where the meridians cross each other twenty-one times, bringing Ch'i into the body. The seven major chakras are placed on the midline of the body, drawing the universal energy into the systems like water going down the plug hole, a vortex of spinning energy feeding into the body from the front and back. The seven main chakra reflexes are found aligned with the spinal reflex and from the top of the thumb to the centre of the base of the palm. Use the tip of your thumb or middle finger to locate the reflexes by lightly scanning the area until a tingling or buzzing sensation can be felt. Make light contact and keep the contact until the sensation ceases. Sometimes a pulse will be felt and again you should maintain contact until the pulsation stops. If there is no pulse, then hold until one is felt. These sensations are thought to indicate hyper or hypofunctioning of a chakra which may eventually result in the malfunction of the corresponding body part. Working on the chakra reflexes 'normalises' their functions as well as working on reflexes of the physical body. In addition, each chakra brings with it an impulse from more subtle levels of our being which affects our endocrine system. The resulting hormonal release is noted by the nervous system and adjustments are made, harmonising the whole.

- ❖ The **crown chakra** relates to the head, autonomic nervous system and endocrine function, and affects our objectivity, emotional maturity, spirituality and natural bodily rhythms. It is linked to the pineal gland and associated diseases are Parkinson's disease, depression, schizophrenia, epilepsy and senile dementia.

- ❖ The **third eye chakra** relates to the skull, brain, eyes, nose and ears, and affects mental states, understanding and vision. Linked to the pituitary gland, associated problems include migraine, glaucoma, cataracts, sinusitis and catarrh.

- ❖ The **throat chakra** relates to the cervical vertebrae, the neck, throat and metabolism, and affects the vocal cords, communication, glandular imbalance, creativity and will. Linked to the thyroid, an imbalance may cause myxoedema, hyperthyroidism, asthma, bronchitis, tonsillitis, tinnitus, anorexia, mouth ulcers and multiple sclerosis.

- ❖ The **heart chakra** relates to the upper thoracic vertebrae, the arms and hands, the heart and the immune system, and affects our ability to feel unconditional love, to empathise and to express our feelings. Its associated gland is the thymus, and associated conditions include heart disease, AIDS and HIV, allergies and cancers.

❖ The **solar plexus chakra** relates to the lower thoracic vertebrae, the stomach, liver, gall bladder, pancreas and spleen, and affects our feelings of self-worth, confidence and ability to get things done. The gland associated with it is the pancreas, and related conditions include diabetes, pancreatitis, liver disease, gall stones, ulcers, hiatus hernia, reflux and coeliac disease.

❖ The **sacral chakra** relates to the lower back, intestines, colon, urinary and lymphatic systems, and affects our relationships, sense of individuality and how we process information. Its related gland is the ovary or testes, imbalances resulting in irritable bowel disease, pre-menstrual problems, fibroids, ovarian cysts, endometriosis, testicular disease and prostate problems.

❖ The **base chakra** relates to the legs and reproductive and skeletal systems, and affects our feelings of belonging and identity, flexibility, patterning and sexuality. It is associated with the adrenal glands and related problems include constipation, piles, colitis, diarrhoea, Crohn's disease, kidney stones, hypo and hypertension, impotence and problems with the joints of the hips, knees and ankles.

As the palm of the hand contains a minor chakra governed by the heart chakra, this point will be covered when working the solar plexus reflex.

## Medical palmistry

Palmistry plays no part in hand reflexology, but palmists during the course of their work have made a number of observations concerning the conditions of the hands and nails, and their relationship to health. These observations may be of use to reflexologists. According to Chinese medical palmistry, which is partly based on Ayurvedic and Buddhist palmistry, each of the five fingers reflects the condition of health at a different age in life. The thumb reflects the condition of health in childhood, the index finger reflects youth, the middle finger shows the condition of health in adult life. The ring finger reflects the health of the later period of adult life and the little finger in old age.

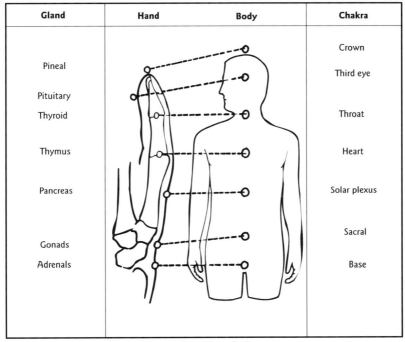

| Gland | Hand | Body | Chakra |
|-------|------|------|--------|

**Figure 5.4: The chakras**

There are five different finger shapes categorised in Chinese medical palmistry:

- ❖ Square: indicates overall good health but with a tendency at times for neurasthenia and kidney or gallstones.
- ❖ Spoon: related to heart and cerebrovascular disease and sometimes diabetes.
- ❖ Cone: with a tendency for disease of the chest.
- ❖ Thin and long: gastrointestinal diseases and depression.
- ❖ Drumstick: indicating possible chronic respiratory diseases and heart or vascular problems.

Strength, length and colour of the fingers would also be significant. On the palms, elevations, colour and condition of the mounds and lines tell the Chinese medical palmist a great deal about the condition of the body, as does the condition of the nails. Observation of the nails and fingers is not exclusive to Eastern traditional medicine; it is used by general practitioners here in the West and also by Indian

Ayurvedic practitioners. Clubbing of the fingers can be observed in people who have respiratory disorders, pale nail beds indicate anaemia and so on. Because the fingernails take between four and six months to grow out, the timing of emotional disturbance or nutritional imbalance can be charted by the position of transverse grooves or dips (*Figure 5.5*).

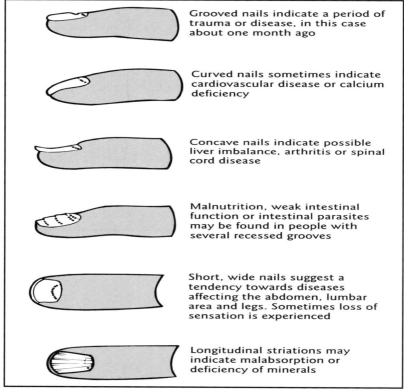

Grooved nails indicate a period of trauma or disease, in this case about one month ago

Curved nails sometimes indicate cardiovascular disease or calcium deficiency

Concave nails indicate possible liver imbalance, arthritis or spinal cord disease

Malnutrition, weak intestinal function or intestinal parasites may be found in people with several recessed grooves

Short, wide nails suggest a tendency towards diseases affecting the abdomen, lumbar area and legs. Sometimes loss of sensation is experienced

Longitudinal striations may indicate malabsorption or deficiency of minerals

**Figure 5.5: Fingernail diagnosis**

## Chinese fingernail diagnosis

While Chinese medical palmistry seeks to identify tendencies towards disease, Chinese fingernail diagnosis seeks to distinguish specific pathologies of the viscera and bowels. As we have seen with the theory of holism, each part of the body is a reflection or miniature of the whole, and so it is with Chinese fingernails diagnosis. When the palm is cupped with the ten fingernails facing each other, the two sets of nails, symmetrical and together echo the homunculus or human fetus (*Figure 5.6*). In this position, the thumbnail represents the head, the index fingernails the chest, back, hands and elbows, the middle fingernails relate to the abdomen and lower back and the ring fingernails to the hips and knees. The feet and ankles correspond to the little fingernails. Ch'i and blood signs on each nail refer to the location, shape, colour of nail and nail-bed markings (*Figure 5.7*).

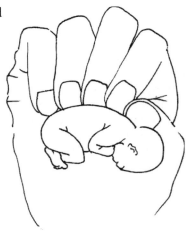

**Figure 5.6: The fingernails reflect the human fetus**

## Metamorphic technique

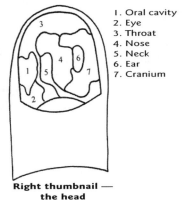

1. Oral cavity
2. Eye
3. Throat
4. Nose
5. Neck
6. Ear
7. Cranium

**Right thumbnail —
the head**

**Figure 5.7: The right thumbnail**

A light and instinctive treatment on the spinal reflexes is more akin to metamorphic technique rather than reflexology, and brings about the type of emotional healing experiences associated with this therapy. Robert St John was a reflexologist searching for a solution to problems arising from conception and prebirth, locked in patterning which affects our physical well-being, outlooks and functioning. His solution was to work on spinal and pelvic reflexes, and in such a way as to be detached from any outcome expectation, working as a catalyst for the patient's innate healing processes. As a result, he was better able to deal with recurring or long-standing problems. Although the metamorphic technique incorporates working on spinal reflexes on the feet, hands and head, I have found that light and detached treatment, on the hands only, initiates clearing responses to conditions such as despondency, anxiety and retrospection which last for two or three days. Following this, there seems to be a feeling of lightness and relief, resulting in clearer and more objective decision-making and clarity of purpose.

## Jin Shin Jyutsu

As a development of acupressure, Jin Shin Jyutsu is a joyful and invaluable tool for self-help and self-knowledge. Again an energy therapy, it works with the rhythms of Ch'i as it circulates up the back of the body and down the front. Seen as the 'battery of life', this energy can be boosted by simple sequences of hand and finger pressure applied to yourself by yourself. If you imagine the body being divided up the middle, there are two sets of twenty-six 'specialist safety energy locks' on each side, left and right; eleven are located on the front and fifteen are on the back. The hands are used as 'jump leads' at these points, boosting the battery and dispersing disharmony in the body, resulting in deep relaxation and a profound sense of well-being. This releases the tensions which cause various physical symptoms and encourages the body to heal more quickly (*Figure 5.8*).

Mental and emotional states can be balanced by holding the fingers and thumbs. Daily application begins a course of self-study in getting to know and help yourself. Holding the fingers and palms also influences the activity of the flow of Ch'i up and down the body. One sequence applied for a few minutes each day encourages us to focus our attitude. All that is needed is a gentle holding of each finger in turn with the palm and fingers of the other hand until you are aware of a pulse. Then move on to the next finger (*Figure 5.9*).

## Aromatherapy

If you are qualified to do so, you may wish to apply essential oils to the hands before or after the treatment, or use massage oils during the treatment. In Ireland, Ogham (pronounced 'Aum') tree oils are applied to the hands according to a Celtic chart. The oils are linked to a very ancient Irish system of healing. Each tree carries its own symbol which is linked to the oil, which in turn can be applied at a particular position on the hand (*Figure 5.9*). A few drops may be rubbed gently into these points on both hands while meditating on its associated symbol, thus acting out a trinity of seeing, being and doing. A few drops of warmed Ogham tree oil of the client's choice is 'healing and soothing'.

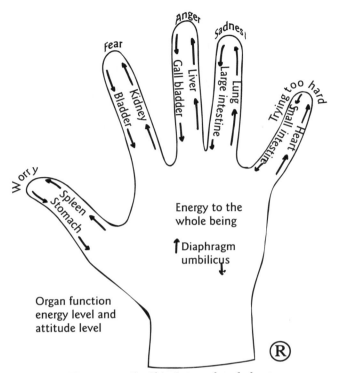

**Figure 5.8: Jin Shin Jyutsu hand chart**

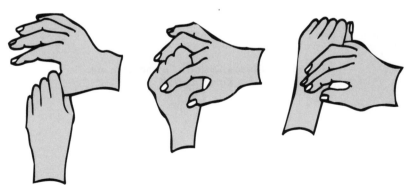

**Figure 5.9: The sequence of Jin Shin Jyutsu grips to relieve worry**

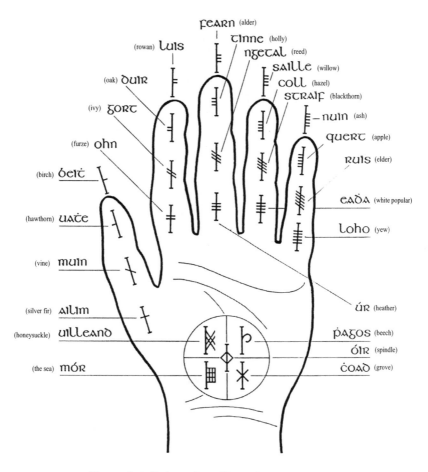

**Figure 5.9: Roison Carroll's Ogham tree oils,**
**© Roisin Carroll**

# 6

## Research, case studies and working notes

This chapter includes:

- case studies
- occasions when hand reflexology is useful
- hands versus feet
- hands and feet together
- referral areas or cross reflexes
- healing crisis
- research.

In the USA foot, hand and ear reflexology are often used together as part of the same treatment session, and hand reflexology is not researched as a separate discipline. One research paper published in *Obstetrics and Gynecology* reported the results obtained from an investigation into premenstrual symptoms (Oleson and Flocco, 1993).

Thirty-five women complaining of previous distress with premenstrual syndrome were randomly assigned to a reflexology treatment group or a placebo group. Twelve formed a control group. All subjects completed a daily diary which monitored thirty-nine premenstrual symptoms on a four-point scale — somatic symptoms, such as sensations of breast tenderness, abdominal bloating and menstrual cramps, and psychological symptoms including mood swings, cravings and confusion. These indicators were recorded each day for two months before treatment, two months during reflexology treatment and two months afterwards. The placebo group received treatment to areas on the hands and feet not considered to be appropriate to the areas relating to premenstrual syndrome.

Analysis of the results demonstrated that there was a significantly greater decrease in premenstrual symptoms for the women given true reflexology treatment than for the women in the placebo group.

In the last few years, much has been done in the way of reflexology research generally, and more specifically on the feet, especially by the Danish Reflexologists Association who have received funding from the Danish Government. Papers include:

### Denmark

1997 Headache and reflexological treatment (Bendstrup and Launsø)

### England

2000 Reflexology and chronic low back pain (Poole)
2000 Does reflexology impact on cancer patients quality of life? (Hodgson)
1998 Reflexology for mental health: a feasibility study in the use of reflexology for community clients with severe and enduring mental illness (Boyd, Evans and Drennen)

Further information can be obtained on these and many other reflexology research papers and pilot studies from the Research Co-ordinator, The Association of Reflexologists, 5 Quantock Lodge, Over Stowey, Bridgewater, Somerset TA5 1HD. The address of the Danish Reflexologists Association Research Committee is: c/o Leila Eriksen, Syvhøjvaenge 268, DK-2625 Vallensbaek, Denmark, tel/fax: +45 4264 8139. The International Council of Reflexologists publishes a Research Analysis Document for $80.00 to include studies from Israel, China and the rest of the world. The contact address is: ICR, PO Box 30513, 10660 Yonge Street, Richmond Hill, Ontario L4C 0C7, Canada.

## Case studies

An eighty-three-year-old man named Edward had enjoyed reflexology after a cataract operation and corneal graft, but had not had treatment for some months. He had a heart attack followed by a triple by-pass operation, after which he was told that his bone marrow would not produce new blood cells and he would need to have regular blood transfusions. He was depressed, irritable, lacking in energy, tired and cold. He suffered from sinus and throat problems and needed to get up several times during the night to relieve himself. He weighed seven stone. After one hand reflexology session, he felt much improved so treatments were given every two or three days for seven sessions. Edward reported that his digestion was 'better than its been for fifty years', and his sinuses were clear for the first time in eighteen months.

Two months later, Edward suffered a mild stroke resulting in loss of sensation and mobility in his left arm. He was banned from driving by his doctor for seven weeks. Hand reflexology was recommended almost immediately on a daily basis. In two days sensation was restored to the tip of the third finger and the numbness in his arm was replaced by a tingling sensation in his fingertips. After three days he was able to dress himself and, after further examinations, his doctor proclaimed him fit to drive. In ten days, Edward felt almost completely back to normal with the added bonus of improved eyesight in the eye that had a corneal implant.

His blood transfusions, however, were imminent, but at his following visit to the hospital it was found that his haemoglobin count had risen from 9g per 100ml to 10.6 g. Six months later this level had dropped a little, but reflexology was resumed and brought the level back up. The transfusions were not necessary. The reflexologist made a special point of working the reflexes to the spleen on the left hand at every opportunity. Edward reports improvement in every way and now weighs nine stone and seven pounds.

Anne had undiagnosed peritonitis which had caused damage to her fallopian tubes. As a result she was offered in-vitro foetal implant in order to conceive, which she tried over a period of eight years and, sadly, was unsuccessful. There was the added problem of her husband having a low sperm count.

Anne had chronic back pain and was a smoker. She had seven hand reflexology treatments, three in the week prior to her eighth IVF attempt. On this occasion, fourteen eggs were produced, the greatest number produced by Anne in any one attempt over her eight years of trying the IVF programme. Seven were fertilised and one egg implanted successfully, resulting in the birth of a healthy girl.

Jane was an NHS chiropodist, unable to work because of the pain caused by a double inguinal hernia, possibly caused by some damage during pregnancy. She had considerable swelling in her right groin and was referred to a specialist in order to be assessed prior to surgery. Jane was raising a small daughter on her own, was overweight, suffered from asthma, some arthritis and tenosynovitis and had a spinal injury seventeen years earlier. She swam and played volleyball regularly when she was able and sought hand reflexology for a volleyball injury which had caused swelling and pain to her right knee.

Jane had five hand reflexology treatments over a period of a month. During this time her knee problem improved and the pain and swelling in her right groin disappeared completely. She was able to resume her work as a chiropodist and quickly resumed her volleyball. When she kept the appointment with the specialist, it was found that surgery was not necessary and Jane has had no further recurrence of this problem.

## Occasions when hand reflexology is useful

Kate is twenty-two years old and suffers from spina bifida, spending most of her days in a wheelchair. She suffers from 'sick headaches', but the frequency and duration have decreased with the use of hand reflexology. She also suffers from painful periods so her reflexologist has shown Kate how to work on her own hands to relieve this pain. Knowing how her headaches have improved, Kate feels confident about the treatment and is pleased to be able to do something positive to help herself.

Peter is in his fifties and has multiple sclerosis. Although almost completely paralysed, he is in good spirits. Hand reflexology for him means regular physical contact in a way acceptable to him. He likes the feeling of 'touch' most of all in his treatment, and enjoys the attention given to him at these sessions.

A lively seven-year-old boy suffering from asthma and eczema thinks foot reflexology is very funny, but loves to work on his own hands as instructed by his therapist. He does this every night before he goes to bed. The reflexologist gave him a chart of the hands and coloured in the areas where he should work. Clinical analysis has shown that when forty-five children between the ages of five months to seven years, and suffering from bronchial asthma, were given reflexology once a day for forty to fifty minutes over a period ranging from two to twelve weeks, clinical symptoms in all forty-five cases disappeared (Duanmu Hui-xian, Health Centre for Women and Children, Haimen, Jiangsu Province).

## Hands versus feet

Foot reflexology is the most popular method of treatment in the UK and if you make an appointment with a reflexologist, this is more likely to be offered to you unless you specify otherwise. There are, however, a number of occasions when hand reflexology would be a more appropriate choice. These are:

- when there is an infection of the feet such as athlete's foot or verruca
- when the foot is injured
- when the feet are so sensitive that any pressure would cause undue discomfort
- when the lower limbs have been amputated
- when access to the feet is restricted, as in the cases of clients in wheelchairs when the legs cannot be raised
- when time is short
- when a client is embarrassed or unwilling to expose his/her feet
- when the client requires discretion, as in a hospital ward
- self-treatment
- homework for clients
- when foot reflexology does not seem to stimulate a healing response or progress has slowed down or stopped.

There are also occasions when hand reflexology can be applied as first aid:

- when seated beside someone in a bus, boat or aeroplane
- when standing or in a confined space
- to comfort someone in a state of shock.

As part of programmes to educate and inform the public, it can be used on the following occasions:

- at health fairs or exhibitions when delegates feel embarrassed about removing their shoes
- to demonstrate reflex points during talks or presentations.

Hand and feet can be worked very well together, especially when things need to be speeded up or there is a time limit or a limit on the number of treatments that can be given.

Some reflexologists have found that better results can be obtained on the hands. Working the web between the thumb and index finger, for example, is particularly useful for working with problems of the large intestines because an acupressure point is in this area. The web can be used consistently for the relief of headaches and migraine headaches, and the fingers for sinus problems. Musculoskeletal problems, such as problems with elbow joints and some spinal conditions, can be dealt with very effectively.

## Hands and feet together

Reflexologists who give treatment to the feet only may find that introducing some hand treatment into the sessions has a number of benefits. It often happens that sensitive points or areas relate more to conditions of the feet rather than sensitive responses of the reflex points themselves, and locating and testing the corresponding points on the hands is a way of checking this. Additional work on the hands at the end of a foot session is a way of reinforcing the foot work and brings speedier results. It is also an opportunity for the client to be involved in self-health, as a short demonstration on the tender points backed by a marked chart encourages the client to work on his/her own hands between treatments and experience the changes in the response for him/herself.

On occasions when the healing process seems to slow down or come to a halt, a hand treatment often breaks the pattern. Treating hands and feet equally during the session is the most balancing way of working, and often the most invigorating for the client. I find that the best approach is:

| | | |
|---|---|---|
| 1 | Opening movements on the feet | = five minutes |
| 2 | Working the left hand | = eight minutes |
| 3 | Working the left foot | = fifteen minutes |
| 4 | Working the right foot | = fifteen minutes |
| 5 | Working the right hand | = eight minutes |
| 6 | Closing movements on the feet | = seven minutes |
| | Total | = fifty-eight minutes |

As it is important to keep the sessions within the hour, this works well, although you may have to learn how to speed up your foot treatment. In my experience, this brisker pace energises clients who are tired and lethargic and, working from left to right as in the sequence described above, wakes them up even more.

If you are going to use hand reflexology to back up your foot treatment, then you may not wish to spend sixteen minutes working the hand. In this case, just a few minutes will do. Work on the points that were found to be sensitive or congested on the feet — just one or two minutes on each point will be sufficient. If the whole foot is sensitive, then you will have to select key points relating to the presenting problem, perhaps working one system, or lightly and quickly covering the whole hand to decrease the sensitivity in the feet. If there is a great deal of pain in the body, select the reflex to this area as a means of effecting pain control.

The hand is the referral area or 'cross reflex' for the foot, so if you wish to work on a condition or injury of the foot itself, you can work on the hand on the corresponding side. Match tarsals with carpals, metatarsals with metacarpals and match each phalange to locate the corresponding reflex. You are working with the zones. If the ankle is injured, you can work on the wrist on the same side and help the ankle to heal. This also corresponds to reflexes of the hips and pelvis. If you cannot work on a big toe, work on the thumb and help the big toe to heal as well as dealing with possible problems in the head and neck. Try working on the hand and the foot at the same time, selecting one point on each.

## Healing crisis

The effects of the body's attempts to cleanse and adjust may result in a number of symptoms that appear to be rather more than the common symptoms of detoxification sometimes experienced after a reflexology treatment — headache, nausea, increase in micturition, diarrhoea or runny nose. At first, it may seem that the treatment is having a detrimental effect on the well-being of the client, but the common experience is that once the symptoms have passed, the client feels a great deal better. The symptoms that manifest may be related to previous illness or trauma, often when these symptoms have been suppressed by drugs. Sometimes it is difficult to tell the difference between the healing reactions and the beginning of a new illness, another reason why taking a medical history is so important. There may be the flu-like symptoms of an aching body, nausea, fatigue, irritability and colds, or pains in the joints, digestive problems or migraine.

The onset of symptoms varies from person to person, sometimes a few hours after a treatment, but more commonly the following day. More severe reactions may continue for two or three days, usually if the treatment is part of a long-term treatment plan and is following a plateau stage when there has been a period of little or no progress. Some reflexologists have reported a deterioration in the condition of clients between the fourth and sixth sessions, followed by much improvement. You may lose your client at this time unless he or she is able to view the symptoms as a positive indication that they are responding to treatment. Although I do not suggest to my clients that they may feel worse following a visit to me, I do make sure that they have my telephone number so that they can call me to discuss any changes in their symptoms. If they do ring, then I can either reassure them that any reactions are normal, or suggest that they visit a general practitioner if I feel something is emerging unrelated to their treatment. People do not expect to feel ill and some people cannot tolerate it at this time, so modify your approach if you think reactions are too severe, or stop seeing them. On the whole, most people feel wonderful after their treatment and the healing crisis is not an issue.

## Conclusion

I hope that this book will enable you to give a confident reflexology treatment and help to develop your reflexology until it becomes your own unique tool. We have differing talents and inclinations and when we have a solid foundation on which to build, we can each begin to make a contribution to reflexology, sharing and exchanging our discoveries. The next few years will, no doubt, bring research which will show how reflexology and other therapies initiate change in physical conditions. We have come into it at a time when its revival is still in its infancy, and can participate in its growth. While we strive to maintain and improve standards in schools of reflexology, carefully nurturing our body of knowledge and taking steps to establish and protect the unique qualities of reflexology, I think we must be generous with our knowledge and allow it to disseminate into other fields.

In *Chapter 5* I have mentioned other therapies in which hands are used to awaken the idea that everything is connected. While we can use reflexology as our ground therapy, we cannot close our minds to the possibility that it may be enhanced by knowledge available in other areas. We should be working with specialists in all fields of healing, both with the medical profession and the alternative therapists. Reflexology is cheap, non-invasive and powerful when properly applied. It has much to offer: it is a delight to give and to receive, and I hope that the joy it brings to you and your clients can match the joy that it has brought to me.

# Reference

Oleson T, Flocco W (1993) Randomized controlled study of premenstrual symptoms treated with ear, hand, and foot reflexology. *Obstet Gynecol* **82**(6): 906–11

# Useful addresses and acknowledgements

My thanks to Roisin Carrroll for her information about the Ogham Tree Oils. More details about these and her workshops can be obtained from:

Roison Carroll
Ogham Apothecary
Carlingford
Co Louth, Ireland

Thanks also to Editha Campbell who is a reflexologist as well as a Jin Shin Jyutsu teacher and practitioner. If you would like to learn Jin Shin Jyutsu, or have a treatment, then contact:

Editha Campbell
40 Archers Road
Eastleigh
Hampshire SO50 9AY

Jin Shin Jyutsu Inc
8719 E San Alberto
Scottsdale, AZ 85258

I am indebted to Hazel Goodwin, Chairman of the Association of Reflexologists, and my teacher, Jane Vukovic for her encouragement. If you would like a reflexology treatment from a qualified practitioner, or a list of courses accredited by the association contact:

The Association of Reflexologists
5 Quantock Lodge
Over Stowey
Bridgewater
Somerset TA5 1HD

The Metamorphic Association
67 Ritherdon Road
Tooting
London SW17 8QE

Lynne Booth
Booth VRT Ltd
Suite 205
60 Westbury Hill
Bristol BS9 3UJ
Tel: 01179 626746
Fax: 01179 626605
e-mail: contact@boothvrt.com
website: www.boothvrt.com

China Reflexology Association
PO Box 2002
Beijing 100026
China

Kristine Walker
e-mail: walkerkristine@hotmail.com

# Further reading

Booth L (2000) *Vertical Reflexology*. Piatkus, London

Issel C (1990) *Reflexology, Art, Science and History*. New Frontier Publishing, Sacramento, CA, USA

Marquardt H (2000) *Reflexotherapy of the Feet*. Thieme, Stuttgart, New York

Page C (1992) *Frontiers of Health: from healing to wholeness*. CW Daniel Company Limited, Saffron Walden

Pitman V, MacKenzie K (1997) *Reflexology. A Practical Approach*. Stanley Thornes, Cheltenham

Vasant L (1984) *Ayurveda, the Science of Self-healing*. Lotus Press, Twin Lakes, Wilmot, WI

Wills P (1995) *The Reflexology Manual*. Headline, London

Xiao-fan Z, Liscum G (1995) *Chinese Medical Palmistry*. Blue Poppy Press, Boulder, CO

# Index